613.2

The New High Protein *Healthy Fast Food* Diet

The New High Protein *Healthy Fast Food* Diet

The effective way to use convenience foods as part of a low-carb diet

Dr Charles & Maureen Clark

Vermilion
LONDON

1 3 5 7 9 10 8 6 4 2

First published in the United Kingdom in 2004 by
Vermilion, an imprint of Ebury Press
Random House UK Ltd
Random House
20 Vauxhall Bridge Road
London SW1V 2SA

Random House Australia (Pty) Limited
20 Alfred Street, Milsons Point, Sydney
New South Wales 2061, Australia

Random House New Zealand Limited
18 Poland Road, Glenfield
Auckland 10, New Zealand

Random House (Pty) Limited
Endulini, 5A Jubilee Road, Parktown 2193, South Africa

Random House UK Limited Reg. No. 954009
www.randomhouse.co.uk
Papers used by Vermilion are natural, recyclable products
made from wood grown in sustainable forests.

A CIP catalogue record for this book is available from the
British Library.

ISBN 0 09 1894786

Typeset by Palimpsest Book Production Limited,
Polmont, Stirlingshire

Printed and bound in Great Britain by
Bookmarque Limited, Croydon, Surrey

Contents

Acknowledgements   vi
Foreword   vii

Introduction   1
Chapter 1   The Essentials of a Successful Healthy
                Diet   5
Chapter 2   Foods Included and Foods Excluded
                From the Diet   33
Chapter 3   The New High Protein Diet
                – Frequently-Asked Questions   45
Chapter 4   How to Prepare Healthy Foods *Quickly*   53
Chapter 5   Breakfast   69
                – Quick and healthy breakfast at home   74
                – Bistro breakfast   104
                – Take-away breakfast   105
Chapter 6   Lunch   111
                – Take-away lunch – cold   117
                – Take-away lunch – hot   132
                – Packed lunch   141
                – Lunch at home   160
                – Bistro lunch   173
Chapter 7   Dinner   177
                – Quick-and-easy dinner at home   181
                – *Really* fast suppers   218
                – Ready-prepared meals   226
                – Restaurant meals   237
Chapter 8   Vegetables and Salads   249
                – Vegetable side-dishes   253
                – Salads   263
Chapter 9   Dressings and Sauces   269
Chapter 10 One Month Meal Plan   277
Chapter 11 Exercise Anywhere!
                The 5-Minute-a-Day Plan   287

Index   305

Acknowledgements

Once again we thank our long-suffering children, David and Heather, for patiently (and sometimes not-so-patiently) trying all the recipes – especially those which did not progress further!

Further information can be obtained on:
www.charlesclark.uk.com

Dr Clark consults at:
The London Diabetic and Lipid Centre
14 Wimpole Street
London
W1G 9SX

Tel.: 020 7636 9901

Foreword

This book has involved considerable research to obtain statistics for the carbohydrate contents of everyday foods present in supermarkets and delicatessens. To ensure accuracy, the nutritional information has been collected from the actual goods themselves where possible, not merely from books and references. All the recipes have been tested (and many others have been discarded) using the best alternatives currently available in supermarkets. The problem of keeping to a low-carbohydrate diet during a hectic lifestyle is recognised by all serious dieters and it is a difficult problem to solve because almost all of the ready-made 'fast' foods available are high-carbohydrate convenience foods. But this book solves that difficult problem in virtually every possible scenario, from take-away food to dinner.

Maureen and I have been involved in medical research for over 20 years. Unlike the popular misconceptions regarding the 'excitement' of research, it usually involves accumulation of facts by a long series of carefully monitored clinical trials. The results of discovering new facts which can be applied in clinical treatment are exciting, but must be applied in a painstaking, considered manner. These principles have been incorporated in this book, which has the potential to significantly impact – in a positive manner – on those members of society most at risk of suffering from the medical effects of an unhealthy, hectic lifestyle. The credit for this immense task should be accorded to Maureen, who suggested the content of the book, performed the vast nutritional research, created most of the recipes and wrote most of the text while I was engaged in the duties of a busy clinical practice.

Introduction

Unfortunately, most people simply don't have the time or the luxury to spend significant amounts of time preparing meals, especially at breakfast or lunch. Whether you are a busy executive or working mum (or both), the hectic pace at which most of us live our lives means that fast food is an integral feature of modern life and it's here to stay. Most of the so-called 'fast foods' contain high proportions of refined carbohydrates and trans fats – the perfect combination to make you fat! But this isn't necessary at all. You can lose weight quickly and easily on a diet comprised mainly of fast 'convenience' foods if you know what to eat, and more importantly, what not to eat. Unlike most other diets, this programme is specifically designed for busy people with busy lifestyles. It allows for virtually every normal situation, from breakfast in a fast-food outlet to dinner in a restaurant, with all the possible permutations of meals and snacks in-between the two extremes.

The aim of this book is to completely change the way you think about food. It will make you realise that you can enjoy all the most delicious foods available, in almost unlimited quantities, and still lose weight and become healthier at the same time. Apart from the immense variety of ready-cooked foods available today – and we will explain the wide choices – you can also cook delicious fresh food in tasty sauces in minutes. You can enjoy sliced beef in oyster sauce in virtually the same time it takes to open tins and packages – a world apart from the usual microwave 'TV dinner'! This book will show you how to enjoy delicious meals in minutes, and hopefully allow you to appreciate how delicious and healthy 'real' food is; the only reason most people eat so-called 'fast' foods is precisely because they are fast, but fresh foods can be just as quick to prepare when you know how.

Most importantly, this programme will allow you to eat healthy and nutritious food while dieting, because it is quite easy to enjoy a healthy, tasty and nutritious diet comprised entirely of 'fast food', although it may not be fast food as you understand the term. In fact, this diet programme is specifically designed to include all the essential nutrients for health. *Every food item has a healthy purpose*, even to the seasoning: you will see that many recipes suggest seasoning with freshly ground black pepper, which not only adds immeasurably to the taste, but also provides a good source of the mineral chromium, essential in the prevention of diabetes.

'Fast food' conjures up images of McDonald's, Kentucky Fried Chicken, Burger King and various other take-away outlets of the same genre. Certainly these *can* be included in a fast food diet if we choose the meals selectively (amazing though this seems) but these types of meals cannot form the basis of any diet. The term 'fast food', as it is used in this book, actually means those foods you can purchase ready-made or those you can prepare quickly and easily. So a real fast food diet is based on quick and easy meals which are also nutritious, because there is no point slimming down to an unhealthy body!

The basis of an effective, healthy diet, on which you are virtually guaranteed to lose weight quickly and painlessly is:

1. It **must** be practical
2. It must eliminate all refined carbohydrates in your diet.
3. It must include a healthy balance of all essential nutrients to promote good health as well as weight loss.
4. Finally, to be successful any diet must be adaptable to virtually every normal everyday situation, without willpower or hunger.

This programme will achieve all the above with *real* fast food: nutritious foods that are ready-prepared, or can be prepared quickly at home. This is certainly not a 'salad and cottage cheese' diet. In fact, nothing could be further from the truth. It includes delicious foods which are healthy and appetising.

The importance of a successful healthy diet is that it must appeal to most of the population, which means that there must be a selection of different types of food. All foods will not appeal to everyone but there is a wide choice of foods to accommodate most tastes. In other words, the diet must suit the dieter, not the other way around, because if you are forced to diet on foods you dislike, or which you cannot easily obtain, your diet will inevitably fail – as all unsuccessful dieters already know. Personally, we find cottage cheese and rice cakes (and other similar 'diet' foods) quite inedible, so this type of food does not appear in this book.

Chapter 1

The Essentials of a Successful Healthy Diet

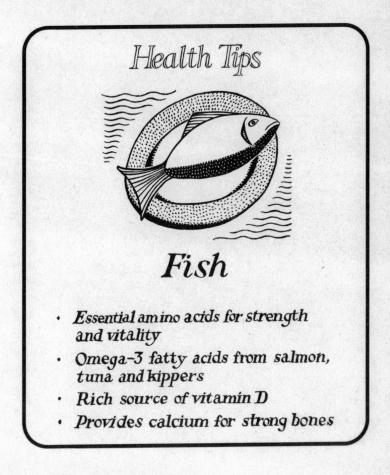

Health Tips

Fish

- *Essential amino acids for strength and vitality*
- *Omega-3 fatty acids from salmon, tuna and kippers*
- *Rich source of vitamin D*
- *Provides calcium for strong bones*

The basis of successful dieting is explained in detail in *The New High Protein Diet* (published by Vermilion), but the basic principles are very simple:

1. The diet must be practical

This basically means that it must fit a busy lifestyle. The meals must either be able to be prepared and cooked quickly, and taste delicious, or the alternative to take-away or restaurant meals must be equally tasty and delicious.

2. The diet must eliminate refined carbohydrates

Essentially, there are two types of diet: either low-calorie or low-carbohydrate.

Low-calorie diets are based on the principle that you consume less calories than you need, so you burn your body fat as energy and become slimmer. On the surface, this seems like common sense, but it is actually completely wrong! It makes the assumption that the body is like a combustion engine consuming fuel. This is far too simplistic. A machine always responds in the same way but the human body is a complex, living organism which responds in different ways to constantly changing situations. Hormones are the 'chemical messengers' which control the smooth functioning of the body, ensuring an even equilibrium and preventing massive swings in all of the millions of chemical reactions which occur every second. They control everything about you, from your moods to the way your body digests food and even to the functioning of the sexual organs.

The hormone which controls the production and breakdown of body fat is 'insulin'. And it is this hormone which absolutely determines whether you will burn your body fat or not. Now to the amazing part: *the amount of insulin you produce is not regulated by the amount of calories you consume.* Insulin production is stimulated by carbohydrates in your diet, not fats or proteins. So if you consume a diet low in carbohydrates, you will programme your body to break down body fat, and if you consume a diet high in carbohydrates, you will not break down body fat efficiently *even if you maintain a low calorie intake.*

So there is absolutely no point in a low-calorie diet. When you lose weight on this type of starvation diet, you are actually losing a significant amount of body protein, which is essential for health. And as very few people can sustain a starvation diet for any length of time, you gain more weight than you originally lost when you return to eating 'normally', as the excess food (usually in the form of carbohydrates) stimulates insulin production to deposit the calories directly as fat!

The diet in this book is a low-carbohydrate diet because that is the only type of diet which will *medically* programme your body to burn body fat as your prime energy source. By eliminating refined carbohydrates from your diet, the amount of insulin in the bloodstream decreases and you stop *making* fat and start *burning* fat. Losing weight really is this simple. No insulin, no fat. This is not a low-calorie or low-fat diet. On the contrary, calories are *virtually unrestricted* on this diet, provided you severely restrict carbohydrates. Calories from proteins and 'healthy fats' (such as extra-virgin olive oil) will not be converted into fat in the absence of carbohydrates. You will not gain weight from the calories in proteins and fats alone, because it is only carbohydrates that stimulate insulin production and it is only insulin that causes calories to be converted into body fat.

The more carbohydrates you consume, the more insulin your body produces. As carbohydrates stimulate insulin production, which programmes your body to make fat (and actually *prevents* your body from breaking down body fat as energy), they are the main reason for obesity, and conditions associated with obesity: heart disease, high blood pressure, diabetes and premature arthritis.

So what exactly are the 'refined' carbohydrates that we have to restrict to ensure successful, painless and sustained weight loss?

- all sugars
- (almost) all bread and flour products
- cakes, pastries, pies and biscuits
- pizza
- rice
- pasta
- cereals
- beer, cider and all sweet and fortified wines (sherry, port)
- sweet drinks (fruit juice and all carbonated drinks except low-calorie 'diet' drinks)
- confectionary, chocolates and sweet desserts

These foods must be eliminated from your diet in the 'weight loss' phase of the diet, but when you have lost sufficient weight and enter the 'weight maintenance' phase, they can be re-introduced *in moderation*.

And to be successful you have to restrict your carbohydrate intake to a maximum of 40–60 grams per day. More than 60 grams per day and insulin production will start to convert the excess calories to body fat; less than 60 grams per day (and preferably less than 40 grams of carbohydrates per day) and insulin will be reduced to such a degree that your body will literally start to burn body fat for energy, even though you are consuming more calories. Without insulin, your body cannot make fat from the calories you consume, and to repeat (because it is essential that you understand this simple process), *the only food that stimulates insulin production is carbohydrates.*

So exactly how difficult is it to keep to less than 60 grams of carbohydrate per day on a diet including *healthy* foods which can either be prepared and cooked relatively quickly or which are easily available ready-prepared? The following is just an example – you certainly do not need to follow this menu – but it explains in very simple terms exactly how easy it is to keep to this diet using widely available nutritious foods which can be quickly prepared.

- Breakfast: ham omelette with mushrooms and tomatoes
- Lunch: prawn mayonnaise open sandwich
- Dinner: lamb rogan josh curry

Total carbohydrates for the day only 39 grams!

Each of the meals is a very large serving (if you wish) and all are prepared in less than 10 minutes, as you will see later in the book. Of course, these are not the only main meals you can enjoy during the day; many other foods with virtually no carbohydrate content can easily be added. You can instantly appreciate how easy – and delicious – a fast food low-carb diet can be, *providing you know what to buy*, and we will provide the immense variety of choices available to you.

But why are some carbohydrates 'bad' and others 'good'. White bread, white pasta and white, polished rice have had almost all of their nutrients removed in the 'refining' process so they essentially consist of pure carbohydrate which is ready to be converted to fat. For example, a typical slice of white bread contains wheat flour, water, yeast, vegetable fat, salt, soya flour, emulsifiers E471 and E481, calcium propionate (to prevent mould growth!), ascorbic acid, E920 and flavourings! There is virtually no nutrition, apart from that added by the manufacturers to comply with legal regulations. And on the loaf of bread from which we are quoting it then states: 'Recommended by nutrition professionals for healthy adults'!

Of course wholemeal bread, pasta and rice are completely different and certainly have significant nutritional value, but they are also high in carbohydrates and must therefore be eliminated during the weight loss phase of the diet. All the nutrients they contain can be obtained from other sources in the diet, so they are certainly not essential.

Because only carbohydrates stimulate insulin production (which converts calories into body fat) *all* carbohydrates must be restricted in our diet. In practice, this means that in addition to *eliminating* the unhealthy refined carbohydrates (above), we must also *restrict* some 'healthy' carbohydrates during the weight loss phase of the diet, which include:

- milk and milk products (the source of the sugar 'lactose')
- fruit (which contains the sugar 'fructose')
- pulses (dried peas and beans)
- starchy vegetables (such as potatoes and parsnips)

These carbohydrates also contain other healthy nutrients, such as proteins, vitamins and minerals, but for the purpose of fat breakdown our body cannot differentiate between 'good' carbohydrates and 'bad' carbohydrates. As insulin (the fat-making hormone) is stimulated by both groups, even healthy, natural carbohydrates must be restricted in the early weight loss phase of the diet. This will have no effect on your health as the vitamins and minerals that these foods contain are all provided by other foods in the diet, so there is no question of the diet lacking any essential nutrients; on the contrary, this diet will include *all* the essential nutrition your body requires, in excess! After you have lost as much weight as you want, these foods can be re-introduced during the weight maintenance part of the diet, since the aim of this diet is to programme your body not just to lose weight quickly, easily and healthily, but also to prevent future weight gain.

Remember, every day you abuse your body with unhealthy food you are accumulating health problems slowly but surely for later in life. If you maintain a diet high in refined carbohydrates for years, your cells gradually become resistant to the effects of insulin and you develop *insulin resistance*. This means that your body makes more and more insulin, which converts the carbohydrates into fat much more quickly, until eventually your body cannot respond to the insulin and the condition called diabetes develops. This is a terrifying scenario as diabetes has many severe complications, such as heart disease, kidney problems and blindness. And this scenario is already happening today: the number of patients developing diabetes is increasing at alarming rates and we are even seeing children developing the adult form of the disease because of a poor diet based on refined carbohydrates. This is even worse when you consider that this type of diabetes is actually preventable: it is largely based on diet, or, more specifically, on a poor diet which is carbohydrate-based. So for many youngsters today, the diet they are following, particularly if there is no exercise to burn off the calories, may well cause their early demise! It really is that serious.

3. The diet must be easy to follow in all situations, without the need for willpower

Basically, if you need strong willpower for a diet then the diet will fail because it definitely does not fit your lifestyle. On the typical low-calorie diet you will probably be eating foods you do not particularly enjoy in quantities that are more suitable for a very small mouse! This is a recipe for disaster. Even if you can sustain this torture for a short time and lose some weight (usually by starvation) you will inevitably regain the weight plus more, because very few people want to live their lives in a constant state of distress – hunger, irritability, poor concentration and constant weakness.

On the contrary, this diet will direct you to easily accessible nutritious foods applicable to virtually every situation – and you will enjoy meals in sufficiently unrestricted quantities so you need never be hungry. By the simple expedient of eliminating refined carbohydrates from your diet, you will be enjoying delicious and nutritious foods in virtually unlimited quantities – and losing body fat at the fastest safe rate for the body (usually 2–3 lbs per week). What could be easier?

4. The diet must include a healthy balance of all essential nutrients to promote good health, as well as weight loss

It is perfectly possible to enjoy a healthy, balanced diet on a programme which restricts refined carbohydrates as there is *virtually no restriction* on healthy foods!

On the contrary, it is virtually impossible to eat a

healthy, balanced diet on a low-calorie regime (which are essentially low-fat diets) because these diets advocate a high intake of carbohydrates, and most refined carbohydrate foods contain virtually no nutrients. So by *reducing* the amount of nutritious foods in your diet (on a low-calorie diet) and by substituting this with refined carbohydrates (like white rice and pasta), which have virtually no nutritional value, nutritional deficiencies are almost inevitable! Even worse, the high levels of carbohydrates in these diets stimulate high insulin levels in the body *which actually prevent you from breaking down body fat*. So not only are you becoming deficient in certain essential vitamins and minerals, but you are consuming the very foods which prevent you losing fat!

In fact, if you embark upon a low-calorie diet, vitamin and mineral deficiencies are *almost inevitable*. And if you follow one failed low-calorie diet with another, which is often the case, your body will gradually become depleted of many essential vitamins and minerals. For example, most low-fat, low-calorie diets specifically restrict cheese and fatty fish (such as sardines, mackerel and herring) because these foods have a relatively high fat content and therefore a relatively high calorie content. Unfortunately, these are the very foods which provide the major sources of vitamin D and calcium in our diet, without which you will develop osteoporosis. Fat is required in the diet to absorb vitamin D and calcium, so if you embark on a low-fat diet you will not absorb these essential nutrients. As a typical example, although skimmed milk and full-cream milk contain similar amounts of calcium, you will only absorb 10% of the calcium from the skimmed milk because fat is required to effectively absorb calcium. This means that you would have to consume 10 litres of skimmed milk to absorb the same amount of calcium as you would obtain from 1 litre of full-cream milk!

In other words, not only is osteoporosis likely on a low-fat, low-calorie diet, it is virtually guaranteed if you maintain this type of unhealthy regime for any significant period. On the other hand, on a low-carbohydrate diet, salmon, sardines, herring, tuna, mackerel and cheese is permitted in *almost unlimited quantities*, so osteoporosis from vitamin D or calcium deficiency is virtually impossible.

Having established that a low-calorie diet is definitely not healthy, what exactly is a healthy 'balanced' diet? The answer is simple: one which contains all the essential nutrients for health – essential proteins, essential fatty acids, vitamins and minerals. Simply including five portions of fruit and vegetables in your diet on a daily basis will not ensure a healthy 'balanced' diet. Although all fresh fruit and vegetables are very nutritious and healthy, there can be significant nutritional deficiencies if the actual nutritional content of the fruit and vegetables is not balanced with the remainder of your diet. For example, there is no significant amount of vitamin B_{12} in fruit and vegetables and vitamin B_{12} is essential for the development of healthy blood cells. This vitamin is essential for health, so it must be obtained from animal sources or supplements.

A healthy, balanced diet must include *all* essential nutrients. This will be achieved on this dietary programme which is specifically designed to include all the nutrients you require. Weight is reduced at the safest healthy rate for the body and when your body reaches its genetically programmed weight, the weight loss will stop. On the contrary, you will probably be consuming the healthiest diet in your life, yet still losing the unhealthy fat that you have accumulated on unhealthy diets based on carbohydrates.

The meals and recipes in this book contain all the

essential nutrients necessary to promote good health. The secret of a healthy diet is to *vary your diet as much as possible*. Do not have the same menu regularly because few meals contain all the essential nutrients for good health. If you can vary your menu, and there are certainly sufficient choices for a very varied diet, you will definitely include all the essential nutrients for good health. In fact, the suggested recipes and meal-plans have been specifically designed to ensure a healthy, truly balanced diet.

Briefly, the essential nutrients you must include in your diet are as follows:

- essential amino acids
- essential fatty acids
- vitamins
- minerals

Essential amino acids are grouped in various combinations to form the different proteins of the body. All the essential amino acids we require are present in all foods of animal origin: beef, lamb, pork, poultry, fish, shellfish and eggs. Most (but not all) the essential amino acids are present in most vegetables and the appropriate combinations of vegetables can ensure that we obtain all the necessary proteins. This diet includes unrestricted animal products and minimal restrictions on vegetables, so there is no possibility of deficiencies of essential amino acids. Extra-lean meat has a saturated fat content of less than 2% which is an almost insignificant amount of saturated fat in the diet.

Essential fatty acids are omega-3 and omega-6 fatty acids. Omega-3 fatty acids are present in the highest concentrations in oily fish (mackerel, sardines, herring, salmon and tuna), eggs and nuts. Omega-6 fatty acids are present in seeds and seed oils, eggs and some vegetables. These are all included – *almost without restriction* – in this diet.

Vitamins are natural chemicals that are present in minute quantities in foods of animal and plant origin. All are incorporated into this diet.

Minerals are natural elements present in foods of animal and plant origin. Once again, this diet has been specifically designed to incorporate all the minerals we require for health.

For those interested, a comprehensive list of essential nutrients and their dietary sources is described in *The New High Protein Diet* and *The Ultimate Diet Counter* (published by Vermilion). A brief review of the relevant chapters will unequivocally demonstrate that all the essential nutrients for health are present in this diet in abundance. The secret is to combine foods in such a manner that the food tastes delicious, is quick and healthy – but also incorporates all essential nutrition with no effort required by the dieter.

5. The diet must not be too expensive

One of the most important issues for most people is finance, for very good reason. Quite simply, to be effective a diet must be economical. We have lost count of the number of recipes which appear in so-called diet plans that advise totally unrealistic ingredients, take hours to prepare and cost a small fortune! One of the most recent advised the reader to have a Waldorf salad for lunch. Apart from the fact that we know of no-one who is able to perform at their peak function following a small salad for lunch, we are also unable to source a Waldorf salad at most of the normal outlets where people have lunch!

We all have many important financial responsibilities and unfortunately food is often the one which is sacrificed first to provide for others. That is a simple fact of life. As this is first and foremost a *practical* book this fact must be taken into account in designing the diet. We are quite lucky in this respect as 'fast food' is usually much more expensive than food which we prepare ourselves; although junk food, like pizzas and pasta, which has virtually no nutrients but merely satisfies our appetites with 'filling' carbohydrates, is relatively inexpensive to purchase and is therefore difficult to compete against on the basis of cost. But from a nutritional aspect, pizzas and pasta are actually relatively expensive! How· can this possibly be true if we all know that pizza and pasta meals are quite cheap? Simply because there is virtually no nutritional value in these meals and the ingredients are very inexpensive so on a weight-for-weight basis, pizza and pasta are actually very expensive.

For example, a typical pizza from the supermarket costs £3–4. The pizza base is essentially just flour and water (costing a few pence) and the topping may be a little (usually *very* little on a commercial pizza) cheese, with either a few slices of pepperoni or ham and is often served with oven-cooked French fries. Total cost £4–5. Total cost of actual ingredients to manufacturer: 20–30 pence maximum. Profit margin: immense. Nutritional value: negligible.

Even worse, if the pizza is purchased from a take-away outlet the cost is usually £8–10, but the cost of ingredients remains relatively negligible.

On the other hand, you could buy 500 grams of salmon fillet – from a supermarket or fishmonger (which could be frozen for later use) – for £4, which can be cooked in a microwave in less than 3 minutes, tastes delicious and is 100% pure essential nutrition. This quantity is easily enough to provide a satisfying meal for four people: with mayonnaise and some stir-fried vegetables (costing less than £2) you have a quick, delicious meal for four in less than 10 minutes for less

than £5! If someone had told you that you could be
enjoying fresh salmon for less cost than frozen pizza –
and in less time than it takes to cook frozen pizza – we
are sure you would not have believed them. But now
you do! Although the prices may change with time, the
relative cost will remain similar, so it is the principle
(rather than the actual prices) which is the main point
of the comparison.

Seemingly expensive meals – like salmon (smoked
or fresh), beef, poultry and shellfish – are actually
not expensive because your appetite is satisfied by
much smaller amounts of food. They can be cooked
quickly (when you know how), taste delicious and
are (with sauces and vegetables) the most nutritious
foods available. You don't *have* to be able to cook to
enjoy quick nutritious meals: we will show you the
easiest and quickest ways of cooking delicious
ingredients in the most cost-effective way. And if you
simply don't want to cook, we will demonstrate how
to buy ready-cooked (or ready-to-cook) food which is
tasty and entirely commensurate with a low-carb
diet. Either way, there is absolutely no reason for
anyone not to be able to diet easily and successfully
– even if they have little time available to cook –
and almost certainly to enjoy healthier food than
ever before!

6. You must *never* allow yourself to be hungry

As a general principle, *never* miss meals, and consume
as much from the permitted foods as you like – it's not
very difficult to keep to this diet! Hunger is one of the
most important reasons for the failure of diets. On a
low-calorie diet, hunger is inevitable as 'you have to eat
less to burn off the fat', or so we are incorrectly
informed by certain 'experts'. Nothing could be further
from the truth! Ninety-five per cent of all low-calorie

diets fail because they are usually based on the worst types of high-carbohydrate foods: cereals, pasta and rice. These are the *same* foods that stimulate the hormone insulin to build fat and to prevent your body from breaking down your body fat. So these diets are medically doomed to failure from the outset.

On this diet you will never be hungry as you can eat virtually unlimited quantities of delicious foods. This removes the temptation to snack on high-carbohydrate foods and as you have medically programmed your body to burn body fat by switching off the high levels of insulin, you burn your own body fat for energy and your weight reduces significantly.

To ensure that you never allow yourself to become hungry between meals, the single most important advice would be to **have a substantial breakfast**.

Breakfast is the most important meal of the day because it literally programmes your body to burn fat (on the correct diet) or build fat (on the wrong diet) for the remainder of the day. It is absolutely essential to have a substantial breakfast of the correct constituents to achieve this aim. This dietary programme will show you how this can be achieved quickly and easily in the morning, either by fast preparation at home or dining out.

Don't worry if you are one of the many people who simply can't eat a satisfying breakfast in the morning. We will explain how to enjoy the correct balance of foods a little later in the day, either prepared quickly at home or pre-purchased, which will achieve the goal of setting your body programme to lose weight easily. This is a *lifestyle* diet, which means that the diet has to be tailored to fit *your* lifestyle, not the other way around. The only inflexible aspect of this diet is the absolute requirement to restrict carbohydrates, because if this is not strictly adhered to, the diet will definitely fail. Apart from this simple restriction, everything else can be tailored accordingly, as you will see.

However any diet will meet with inevitable disaster if you have no breakfast, then snack on high carbohydrate foods (like biscuits or pastries) later in the morning, just because your low blood sugar levels need to be restored.

7. You *must* plan ahead

The secret of successful dieting is successful shopping. You have to keep a stock of certain foods available or, when you become hungry, you will inevitably snack on the high-carbohydrate foods which are instantly available, such as chocolate, potato crisps, crackers and biscuits. And the importance of shopping is not only what you buy, but equally importantly, what you *don't* buy. Do not have cakes, biscuits, chocolate, potato crisps, rice, pasta and white bread available, and then you can be absolutely certain that you will never ruin your diet by consuming these nutritionally disastrous foods!

Apart from the situation at home, you must also have a daily plan of *where* you intend to have breakfast, lunch and dinner, and how these choices will fit in with your diet. For example, you may decide to have breakfast at home, lunch from a take-away sandwich delicatessen and dinner in a restaurant. Plan your dietary programme the previous day and your diet is guaranteed to be successful. It will only take a few minutes and will prevent the need for carbohydrate snacking during the day.

8. *You* must really want to lose fat!

This seems obvious but it's not. It means that you can't go into any diet and expect it to be successful unless you intend to keep to the rules. Obviously there is a responsibility on the diet to make sure that the rules are practical and sensible (i.e. not starvation!) It is certainly unreasonable (in our opinion) to expect anyone to starve themselves on a daily basis while trying to carry out all the responsibilities of work and looking after a family, then blame *them* when the diet fails, as it inevitably will. No 'normal' human being can sustain constant hunger and irritability and still perform to their optimal function! On this diet you will enjoy almost unlimited quantities of delicious foods which are either widely available or are quick and easy to prepare, so that hunger and willpower are definitely not necessary on this programme. But, you still need to really *want* to lose your body fat, not just weight, because it is actually the body fat that you *will* lose on this diet.

9. Learn to think laterally about food

Don't be trapped into eating the same old carbohydrates in meals just because they're always prepared that way. For example, you don't *have* to have curry with rice. The rice has virtually no flavour (especially white rice), it merely provides the 'filler' for the curry and because it is almost pure carbohydrate it makes the meal very fattening indeed! In fact, it is simple to enjoy home-made or commercially-prepared curries which are very low in carbohydrates (the fattening part) providing you substitute the rice with a low-carbohydrate alternative, such as ready-prepared watercress and rocket salad, or stir-fried peppers and courgettes: infinitely healthier and tastier than plain old rice.

Similarly, delicious Italian sauces do not have to accompany pasta. There is hardly any carbohydrate in a Bolognaise sauce with lean mince, tomatoes, onions, garlic and oregano so why not enjoy it with mangetout and French beans? Purchased ready-prepared, these vegetables cook in less than 3 minutes in a microwave oven, are packed with essential nutrients and accompany a spicy, meaty Bolognaise sauce perfectly.

Don't be caught in the carbohydrate food trap. Think of other food combinations and enjoy them. The only reason that refined carbohydrates are always paired with the real food is that carbohydrates are fillers – nothing more – satisfying appetite but providing little nutrition.

10. Everyone can cook delicious, healthy meals easily!

You may be one of those people who think they can't cook, and therefore don't want to cook because they can't cook. This book will teach the most ardent anticook fan that they can cook easily in minutes with no more effort than switching on the microwave oven and turning on the cooker. How can we be so certain? Surely that is a ridiculous statement? Certainly not! If you can switch on a microwave oven you can enjoy a delicious meal in minutes. No, not one of the microwave takeaway dinners, but real food! Easily proved: place two salmon fillets in a microwave container, cover and cook on 'high' for 2½ minutes and allow to stand for a further minute. At the same time, heat 50 grams of butter in a small saucepan until melted, stir in 1 tablespoon of lemon juice and serve the lemon butter sauce you have just prepared over the salmon fillet with a pre-washed salad of watercress and rocket. The whole meal took less than 4 minutes, tastes divine and is incredibly nutritious. And we defy even the most die-hard bachelor to be unable to switch on the microwave oven!

11. Read the label on packaged foods

Many foods contain 'hidden' sugars and other carbohydrates. On packaged foods (plastic, tins, jars) there is almost always a label detailing the nutritional content of the food. Below is a typical example from a supermarket packaged curry.

Typical Values	Nutrition per 100 g	per Pack
Energy kJ	455	1595
kcal	110	385
Protein g	11.3	39.6
Carbohydrate g	(4.1)	(14.4)
of which sugars g	1.5	5.3
Fat g	5.2	18.2
of which saturates g	0.6	2.1
Fibre g	1.2	4.2
Sodium g	0.36	1.26
Equivalent as salt **g**	0.9	3.2

It all looks very complicated but, of course, it isn't. As with most seemingly complicated information there is usually a simple solution. The only information you need is the carbohydrate content (circled above). Look for the carbohydrate content per 100 g and per pack. If it is more than 7 g per 100 grams it is probably going to be too high in carbohydrates for your diet unless you intend only having a little. For example, chocolate contains about 60 grams of carbohydrate per 100 grams!

If you intend to divide the contents of the package (plastic, jar, tin) between several people, simply divide the total carbohydrate content per pack by the number of people and you have the carbohydrate content per person. You can see from this example that if you were to eat this entire curry yourself you would only be incurring 14 grams of carbohydrate, which is relatively little for an entire meal. And the saturated fat content is only 0.6 grams per 100 grams – virtually insignificant.

12. Have the correct kitchen equipment

Having the 'correct' kitchen equipment does not involve considerable expense or inconvenience. This certainly does not require you to purchase equipment that is out of the ordinary like deep fat fryers or complicated blenders, none of which are necessary or desirable for most good cooking anyway. But there are a few items of equipment – most of which are present in the average kitchen – that will definitely assist the production of quick healthy meals for your low-carb diet:

a. Wok or large frying pan: essential for stir-frying.

b. Large saucepan or steamer: essential for steaming vegetables.

c. Microwave oven: not essential, but will undoubtedly accelerate the cooking of many standard meals, especially breakfast.

d. Microwave cookware: again not essential, but the correct cookware for different microwaved meals ensures success. As microwave cookware is made of plastic and very inexpensive, this will cause no significant financial burden.

e. Crêpe-maker: definitely not essential, but very useful if you like crêpes, which are a very versatile meal. Again, this piece of equipment is not expensive

And apart from the standard utensils and equipment you would expect in the average kitchen (and most of the above would be present in the average kitchen) this is really all you would require for guaranteed success with the recipes in this diet.

13. Microwave cooking – the ultimate solution

It is not necessary to own a microwave oven to follow this diet as all meals can be prepared by a quick traditional method. However, if you do have access to a microwave then you will soon realise how versatile it really is and how delicious meals – from breakfast to dinner – can be prepared in minutes. But this is not microwave cooking as you probably perceive it. It is not about placing a packet of food (of usually dubious nutritional value and even less taste) in the microwave but rather using *real* food (like fresh fish, meat, eggs and vegetables) and enjoying delicious and healthy meals within minutes. And the exciting part is that *anyone can cook using a microwave oven!* The days of following complex recipes with complicated cooking techniques are over. Anyone can lay a fillet of fish in a microwave-safe dish, place it in the microwave and (depending on the power of the microwave) set the timer for 2–3 minutes. The fish is cooked to perfection and tastes delicious, and as an added bonus, you are enjoying a successful weight-loss programme which just happens to be quick and simple (and actually much less expensive than the so-called proprietary 'diet foods'.)

Before we commence, it is probably advisable to explain how the microwave oven works and what it can (and can't) do, because there seem to be more myths about microwave cooking than just about any other single topic in cookery.

Microwaves are waves of energy which are produced within the oven. The energy is contained in the oven and, contrary to popular belief, does not leak out. How can we be so sure? Simply because the door to the microwave oven has emergency cut-off switches which switch off the power if the seal is broken (by opening the door). Unlike conventional cooking where the food is heated from the outside, in a microwave oven there is no external heat: the water in the food absorbs the energy waves, converting them into heat which cooks the food. Because most of the heat is actually generated *within* the food there is very little wastage of energy and most foods cook much more quickly (and more inexpensively) than in a conventional oven. The other advantage, of course, is that the food is cooking *without supervision*, so you can be busy elsewhere during the cooking process. But a word of caution: you have to remove the food from the microwave and open the container within a minute of the cooking process having completed as *the food continues to cook in its own heat after the microwave timer has switched off the oven.* So don't forget about the meal or it will be overcooked. The simple way to avoid this is to cook the meal just as you are ready to eat as it usually only takes a few minutes.

What a microwave oven can do

- Cook most foods quickly – usually in a quarter of the time needed by conventional methods – so is ideal for the busy cook.
- Cook safely without supervision.
- Retain most of the nutrients (and flavour) of the food.
- Cook food easily without the need for complex cooking skills.
- Cook *cleanly*: in other words, usually only one or two dishes are required to cook an entire meal, so you save time on washing up!
- Thaw food – once again, ideal for those moments when you have forgotten to take the evening meal out of the freezer!

And if all the above were not enough to convince you

of the advantages of microwave cooking, it's usually much less expensive (in energy) than conventional cooking and so it saves you money!

However, let's not get carried away. There are many things a microwave can do better than conventional methods, but there are also some that it can't do very well.

What a microwave oven *can't* do

- Cook eggs in their shells. However it cooks eggs virtually every other way much better (and more cleanly) than the conventional methods: fried, scrambled, poached and omelette. Having said that, microwave ovens *can* cook boiled eggs *but only using a specific microwave egg-boiling container* which is commercially available and is inexpensive.

- Brown or toast food (unless it has a conventional convection oven facility), so you don't have the brown crispy effect of the conventional roast.

- Impart the same mixture of flavours that stir-frying can achieve for certain meals.

- Cook pasta, rice or pulses faster than conventional methods, but as these are the very foods which are *excluded* from a low-carb diet, this restriction needn't be an issue.

The other major advantage of microwave cooking is that the containers required are usually plastic and very inexpensive, so the start-up costs are very low and the ongoing costs are virtually non-existent. It is worthwhile investing in specifically designed microwave cookware of the correct shape for individual types of food because the improvement in the results of cooking are incredible. Typical examples of microwave cookware which are custom-designed for specific types of cooking include:

- Triple cooker: a triple-layered microwave cooking dish that allows you to cook the complete meal at once. For example, meat is initially cooked in the lowest layer, then the vegetable layer is added to allow the vegetables to steam. Chicken casserole with green vegetables is ready in less than 20 minutes using this method.

- Microwave wok: stir-fried meals cook in 8–10 minutes.

- Microwave fish steamer: fillets of haddock, cod, salmon, trout and plaice cook to perfection in 3–4 minutes.

- Egg poacher, egg boiler, omelette maker: all specifically designed to cook eggs perfectly in less than 3 minutes.

- Bacon cooker: cooks bacon to perfection in 3–4 minutes, even crispy bacon!

- Burger maker: you can even enjoy your favourite burger recipe with a no supervision approach. The burger will cook in 3 minutes, without the need for turning.

Many of the recipes in the book provide a microwave method of cooking which, in all cases described, is much quicker and simpler than the conventional technique. This is particularly useful at breakfast where virtually all standard cooked breakfasts – including bacon and eggs – can be cooked in less than 5 minutes *without supervision*.

A word of caution! Microwave ovens vary in power, usually from 650 to 900 watts. **The cooking times for the recipes in this book refer to an 850 watt oven:** if you have an 600–700 watt microwave, increase the cooking time by about 33%. As each oven varies slightly from another, the cooking times are approximate only. You have to become accustomed to your own oven and experiment to discover the correct time. The easiest way is to cook the meal for slightly less than the recommended time, check to see the state of cooking, and return the meal to the microwave for another 30–40 seconds. After a few meals, you will soon know the power of your oven fairly accurately. Remember that cooking continues *after* the microwave has switched off, as the food cooks in its own heat, so you have to remove the food from the container within a minute after the timer has stopped or the food will be overcooked.

In summary, the principles on which this diet is based could not be simpler:

- It is practical for 'normal' living.
- All refined carbohydrates are severely restricted.
- The diet includes a healthy balance of all essential nutrients to promote good health, as well as weight loss.
- Easy to follow in all situations, without the need for willpower.
- Relatively inexpensive.

And there are several simple requirements of the dieter on this programme:

- You must *never* allow yourself to be hungry.
- You *must* plan ahead.
- You must really want to lose fat!
- Learn to *think laterally* about food.

- Realise that *everyone* – however seemingly inexperienced in cooking – can cook delicious and healthy meals easily!
- Read the label on packaged foods.
- Have the correct kitchen equipment.

On the basis of these simple principles you will actually enjoy losing weight and feeling healthier. There will be no willpower needed, as there is no hunger and no tasteless meals. And, this can all be achieved on a diet composed of *real* food which can be tailored to any lifestyle. The only requirement is that you really *want* to lose weight. If you do, success is guaranteed.

Chapter 2

Foods Included and Foods Excluded From the Diet

The general guidelines for a successful diet are explained in detail in our previous books, *The New High Protein Diet*, *The New High Protein Diet Cookbook* and *The Ultimate Diet Counter*, but it is essential to reiterate the principles of the diet as they form the basis of all that follows.

The essential rule of the diet is that you must restrict carbohydrates to 40–60 grams per day. The best way of keeping within the carbohydrate limit is to refer to *The Ultimate Diet Counter*, which will give you a quick and simple answer to the carbohydrate content of all groups of foods. Follow these simple guidelines and you will easily keep to the restriction of carbohydrates.

Virtually unrestricted foods

- Virtually no restriction on the amount of protein: beef, lamb, pork, poultry, fish and shellfish. Keep to extra-lean meats as these have less than 2% saturated fat content.
- Virtually no restriction on 'pure' fats.
- Fresh vegetables – except potatoes, parsnips and carrots.
- Eggs (up to two per day) – providing you like eggs!
- Alcohol: dry wine (white or red) and spirits, in moderation.
- Tea.
- 'Diet' soft drinks.

Foods to be avoided

- Carbohydrates <u>must</u> be severely restricted to a maximum of 40-60 grams per day, which effectively means no bread, pasta, rice, pies, cakes, biscuits or confectionary.

- Fruit – one piece per day (not bananas!).
- Alcohol: no beer, cider or fortified/sweet wines (sherry, port, Madeira).
- Coffee – or at least drink decaffeinated.
- Milk – even skimmed milk – except a little in tea/coffee.
- Fresh fruit juices.
- Pulses or grains (in the early stage of the diet only).
- Carbonated soft drinks, except the 'diet' variety.

General advice

- Stir-fry, steam or microwave food as much as possible.
- Incorporate garlic and ginger into your diet.
- Eat a substantial breakfast.
- Eat an orange (or take a vitamin C supplement) every day.
- Include herbs and spices in your diet.
- Multivitamin supplements – one per day.
- Exercise – walking and isometric exercise (see pages 287–303).
- Measure shape before weight. Fat is half the weight of protein so you'll lose the centimetres (or inches) from your waist and hips faster than the kilos (or pounds).
- Vary your menu as much as possible.

The basis of a successful and healthy diet is explained in Chapter 1 and the general rules of the diet are explained above, but now we have to specify exactly which foods you can include in your diet (in virtually unlimited quantities) and those you can't. This diet is the opposite of the low-calorie diet: on this diet you can eat virtually as many calories as you want (because you won't be counting calories) but you must exclude certain foods for the diet to be successful. This is not a forgiving diet: if you exceed the limit of 60 grams of carbohydrate per day (or, preferably, 40 grams) you will increase your insulin levels to the level that will convert all the calories in your diet (from fat and protein) into body fat. However, providing you restrict your carbohydrate intake to less than the permitted maximum of 60 grams, you can enjoy virtually unlimited calories and still lose weight because the hormone that converts calories into body fat – insulin – has been switched off.

The other important reason to maintain a low-carbohydrate intake is that refined carbohydrates have an addictive effect: the more you eat, the more you want to eat. By reducing your intake of carbohydrates, the insulin level decreases *and the addiction is removed*. In other words, after a few weeks on this diet, you will no longer have the *desire* to consume large quantities of refined carbohydrates, so the diet is really self-sustaining: the longer you restrict refined carbohydrates, the easier it becomes. So you can appreciate that the occasional chocolate bar will ruin your diet, not only because it exceeds the carbohydrate daily limit, but also because it maintains your addiction to carbohydrates. To gain the benefits of enjoying virtually unlimited quantities of other foods, refined carbohydrates *must* be severely restricted initially.

The following is a simple guide to foods included or excluded from the diet.

Foods included virtually without restriction

Fish and shellfish
Poultry
Meat – especially extra-lean meat
Vegetables (except those with a high-carbohydrate content, such as potatoes, carrots and parsnips)
Oils and dressings

Sauces

Herbs and spices

Foods where some restrictions apply

Drinks

Dairy products

Eggs (up to two per day)

Fruit

Nuts

Soups

Foods excluded during the weight loss phase

Biscuits, cakes and pastries

Bread, flour, grains and cereals

Desserts

Fast foods

Pasta and noodles

Rice

Snack foods

We are now going to show you how, with just a little planning and forethought, these lists can be used in a diet which can be applied to virtually any situation. They will form the basis of successful and healthy dieting. Providing you understand and adhere to these simple principles, you will instantly know which convenience foods are included and which you must completely avoid.

As a simple example, you can have a quarter-pounder burger at McDonald's, providing you leave the bun. Eat the filling (which is virtually carbohydrate-free) and leave the bun (which is virtually pure carbohydrate) and you will continue to diet successfully. Of course, we are certainly not recommending that you patronise McDonald's, it is merely a demonstration that even the most famous of 'fast' foods have some redeeming and healthy features.

The secret of successful dieting is planning. You *must*

maintain a reasonable stock of certain essential foods in your kitchen to ensure the success of a diet because, if you don't have the ingredients for a healthy meal instantly available, you will inevitably return to our old enemies the refined carbohydrates and trans fats. Keep a stock of the following (fairly simple) essential foods and you can be sure of success. They may seem a little expensive at the beginning of the diet, but many of the ingredients (such as herbs and oils) will last a long time and are actually quite inexpensive in the long term. In fact, you will find that the food you are eating will be of a far higher standard but actually less expensive than pre-packaged, high-carbohydrate foods, because you will consume smaller portions *naturally*. Foods rich in essential fats and proteins *naturally* satisfy an appetite, unlike foods composed of refined sugars and fats, which do not satisfy the appetite and therefore cause you to eat much more because you are hungry for longer.

These ingredients form the basis of many meals which can be quickly prepared at home and, most importantly, they form the basis of a *healthy* diet which can be easily maintained despite the most hectic of lifestyles. All are widely available, and none is horrendously expensive. Unless you maintain a stock of basic ingredients which can be instantly combined for quick, healthy (and delicious) meals, you will inevitably snack on high-carbohydrate convenience foods and your diet will fail (along with your health!).

You don't even need to shop yourself! If you are too busy, simply shop online. All major supermarkets offer an online shopping and delivery service: keep a list of the stock items (described below) and top up the list as and when necessary. It will only take a few minutes per week to check your supply of stock items and you will then be sure of always being able to keep to the diet. This diet really can be adapted to all lifestyles providing you are serious in your intention to lose weight.

At one time or another everyone has the problem of preparing a supper in 10–15 minutes after a very tiring day. Some of us unfortunately have that problem most days of the week! A properly stocked kitchen will prevent the necessity of ruining the diet with the ever-ready quick-fix carbohydrates. For example, always having a supply of eggs, milk, onions, tomatoes and preferably, but not essentially, some fresh basil or parsley means that you can prepare a delicious meal of scrambled eggs (or omelette) with onions, tomatoes, basil or parsley in less than 3 minutes in a microwave oven, and only slightly longer using a traditional method of cooking: even faster than the typical microwavable 'TV dinner', and infinitely more healthy. The following are essential items to stock (obviously omitting any foods you don't like).

Vegetables and Salads

Go into the vegetable section of your local supermarket and actually look at the selection available. In addition to the standard vegetables there is also a wide selection of prepared vegetables, usually washed and chopped (if appropriate to the vegetable) in plastic packages. This includes mangetout, carrots, peas, French beans, sugarsnap peas, spinach leaves, asparagus, curly kale, cauliflower and broccoli. And there is a very wide selection of mixed salad leaves: rocket, watercress, various mixtures of lettuce leaves and herbs. These are all ideally suited to the cook in a hurry. In effect, they are healthy 'fast' foods which can be cooked – without supervision – in a microwave in minutes (as we will describe later).

Whilst you certainly don't need to keep a stock of all these various ingredients at the same time, always have some prepared vegetables or salads available and you can be certain of enjoying a healthy and delicious meal at short notice. Many of the recipes have been specifically designed to incorporate vegetables which are available ready-prepared to enable you to keep to your healthy diet even though you have little time for food preparation.

- ready-prepared vegetables e.g. stir-fry
- pre-washed and trimmed mangetout, French beans, carrots, broccoli, curly kale and sugarsnap peas
- ready-prepared salads of various combinations: watercress, watercress and rocket, spinach (or baby spinach) leaves and mixed herbs

The following vegetables and herbs are *absolutely* essential, and you should make sure you always have a stock available.

- garlic
- onions (preferably red or brown)
- herbs (fresh if possible): basil, coriander, flat-leaf parsley, chives and dill
  or, if not possible, keep a supply of dried herbs: basil, coriander, thyme and rosemary
- fresh root ginger
- fresh tomatoes (preferably on-the-vine)
- tinned tomatoes (preferably plum tomatoes)
- tomato purée
- a stock of fresh vegetables, especially red and yellow peppers, kale, spring onions, mangetout, French beans and sugersnap peas (see above)

Oils, Dressings and Sauces

- extra-virgin olive oil (absolutely essential)
- groundnut oil (providing you are not allergic to nuts)
- sesame oil
- white wine vinegar
- balsamic vinegar

41

- mayonnaise
- crème fraîche (on occasions)
- sour cream (on occasions)
- butter
- oyster sauce
- chilli sauce
- mustard: Dijon and wholegrain
- various ready-prepared stocks: beef, chicken, fish and vegetable. There are many excellent stocks available, but always keep a supply of stock cubes ready for those times when you run out (which is guaranteed to happen!)

Cheese

- Always have at least one (and preferably two) cheeses available. This is obviously dependent on individual taste, but Emmental, Gruyere, Gouda and Edam are particularly useful as they melt very easily in cooking

Eggs

- Unless you don't like eggs, *always* keep a good supply of fresh, large, free-range eggs available. They are very healthy, and can always provide a delicious meal quickly – thereby preventing you from falling for the quick high-carb 'fix'

Fresh beef, poultry, pork or lamb

- Once again, you don't have to keep a stock of all of these, but always have fresh meat or poultry available. This is relatively easy with a freezer, and makes the difference between a diet being successful or failing because of lack of ingredients

Fish

- Eat fresh fish at least once a week – easily

purchased during the weekly shopping. If you don't have time to shop every week it can be frozen for later use. Fish figures prominently in this book as it is the ultimate healthy fast food. Packed with healthy nutrients, from essential amino acids to essential fatty acids, the immense variety of fish and shellfish means that you have an almost infinite variety of possible meals. And although we have described many delicious accompaniments to fish, it is delicious alone, with perhaps just some seasoning and a sprinkle of lemon juice

- Tinned tuna and salmon. Absolutely essential. Packed with nutrients (especially vitamin D, calcium and omega-3 essential fatty acids). With tuna available you can always be certain of a swift and delicious supper in minutes. Tuna must be packed in brine or freshwater as the oil can spoil the complementary flavours you add to recipes
- Shellfish, preferably fresh (which usually last two to three days) but frozen prawns if all else fails

Spices

- Essential dried spices are cumin, turmeric, chilli, paprika, garam masala and cinnamon. Despite the antipathy of purists, you have to keep a medium curry powder available to create delicious curries *quickly*, because often there simply is not enough time to prepare the curry mixture from scratch
- Whole peppercorns are another essential. Invest in a peppergrinder for maximum flavour and health-giving properties

Fruit

- Fruit is restricted in the initial weight loss phase of the diet, but always keep a supply of oranges, lemons or limes available as these are regularly added to meals for added zest (and vitamin C)

Nuts and Seeds

- Excellent as delicious, healthy snacks
- Nuts suitable for a low-carb diet include walnuts, pine nuts and Brazils. Nuts to avoid (or very severely restrict) are cashews and sweet chestnuts
- Seeds for snacks (and omega-6 essential fatty acids) are sunflower seeds
- Seeds for stir-fries are sesame seeds

This list may seem expensive at first, but it isn't really. You don't need all of the ingredients at once, but remember most (like herbs and spices) will last through many meals and these foods are *replacing* those you normally eat, so the cost factor is negligible in the long term. And you are not only losing weight quickly, but also becoming healthier on this diet!

Chapter 3

The New High Protein Diet –
Frequently-Asked Questions

There are several questions about *The New High Protein Diet* which are asked so frequently that it would be prudent to dispel some of the myths and fantasies that seem to surround this form of low-carb diet. In all fairness, many of these myths and fantasies have been deliberately propagated by some members of the diet industry who, quite frankly, should know better!

How does the New High Protein Diet differ from the Atkins Diet?

This is definitely the most frequently asked question. Essentially both diets are low-carbohydrate diets but there the resemblance ends.

The Atkins Diet advises a carbohydrate restriction of less than 20 grams per day in the induction phase, which is really quite severe. This involves restriction of all carbohydrates, including vegetables. As it is not possible to obtain all of the essential nutrients which the body needs on this regime, the Atkins Diet recommends taking dietary supplements.

The New High Protein Diet advises much less restriction on carbohydrates (40–60 grams per day) which is not only easier to maintain, it allows all essential nutrients to be obtained from your diet because virtually all vegetables are unrestricted. The restriction is almost exclusively confined to refined carbohydrates only: bread, pasta, rice, cakes, biscuits and confectionary. The only 'healthy' foods which are restricted (and only in the weight loss phase of the diet) are milk, pulses, wholegrains and fruit. Most vegetables are unrestricted; the only exceptions are the high-carbohydrate root vegetables such as potatoes and parsnips. The New High Protein Diet is specifically designed to provide *all* the essential proteins, fatty acids, vitamins and minerals which we need for health. Although it advises taking a single multivitamin supplement tablet daily, that is only a safety precaution for individuals who may not follow the prescribed regime; if you follow the guidelines you will obtain all of the necessary nutrients – in abundance – without supplements.

Isn't too much protein unhealthy?

No it is not. In actual fact you are not really consuming much more protein than previously! How can this be correct if it is a 'high-protein' diet? Because you consume more protein as a *proportion* of your diet rather than more protein as an *amount*. Let us demonstrate how a high-protein diet does not necessarily involve consuming more protein. For example, if every 100 grams of food in your diet comprises 30 grams protein, 30 grams fat and 40 grams carbohydrate, the protein component would constitute 30% of the diet. If you omit the carbohydrate component, there is still only 30 grams of protein but the *proportion* of protein which this constitutes is 50% of the diet i.e. 30 grams protein in a 60 gram meal.

Omitting refined carbohydrates from your diet does not necessarily result in consuming more fats and proteins. On the contrary, fats and protein foods satisfy hunger quickly and you will find that your appetite is satisfied with less food. So you can now understand how a high-protein diet may not necessarily entail consuming more protein because it is the amount of protein as a *proportion* of your diet *rather than the actual amount* in your diet.

This is also the explanation of how we can allow virtually unlimited amounts of pure proteins and fats in your diet because we know that these foods satisfy hunger much better than carbohydrates. Therefore your appetite will *naturally* be satisfied with less food and you will inevitably consume less.

How can I be sure I am obtaining all the nutrients I need to stay healthy on this diet?
The New High Protein Diet has been specifically designed to ensure that *all* the essential nutrients – amino acids, essential fatty acids, vitamins and minerals – are present in abundance. There is no counting of calories and, providing you severely restrict refined carbohydrates, there is virtually no other restriction on the amounts of other foods you can enjoy. And, as refined carbohydrates have *virtually no intrinsic nutritional value whatsoever* (apart from certain additives), it is obvious that all other foods contain the essential nutrition for health. There is a section in the companion book (*The Ultimate Diet Counter*) which describes all the essential nutrients we require for health and it also explains how these essential nutrients are provided by this diet.

Once again, as a comparison, it is virtually impossible to obtain all of these essential nutrients for health on a low-calorie or low-fat diet because these are essentially starvation diets where you are consuming *less* than you require. If this is continued on a long-term basis malnutrition of certain essential nutrients is inevitable.

Don't high protein diets damage the kidneys?
No. Simple straightforward answer. This is a myth commonly proposed by some dietitians and other so-called experts to discredit high protein diets. In medical terms, the kidneys remove protein waste products from our bodies which are then passed out of the body in the urine. If you have kidney disease, which is a very serious condition, then too much protein would be detrimental to your health. But

kidney disease is a very serious health problem and *any diet would be dangerous in these circumstances*. In other words, if you have kidney disease you should not commence a diet of any nature.

Does the New High Protein Diet cause osteoporosis?

No. In fact it would be impossible to develop osteoporosis on the New High Protein Diet. Osteoporosis is a deficiency disease, the main cause of which is a deficiency of vitamin D and calcium in the diet. The main dietary sources of vitamin D and calcium are fatty fish (such as herring, mackerel, sardines, tuna and salmon), dairy products, cheese and eggs. On the New High Protein Diet, apart from a slight restriction of milk intake, these are the foods which you are actually encouraged to include in your diet, so you can see it is impossible to develop a malnutrition of vitamin D and calcium on this diet.

On the other hand, these are the very foods which are *severely restricted* on a low-calorie or low-fat diet because they are high in calories. So any prolonged low-fat or low-calorie diet is likely to cause osteoporosis, certainly not the New High Protein Diet.

Will I be eating too much fat on this diet?

Once again the answer is 'no'. This is not a high-fat diet. In fact it simply is not possible to consume too much 'pure' fat in your diet because natural foods which have a higher fat content and a very low carbohydrate content (such as cheese, cream, eggs, salmon and mackerel) satisfy hunger very successfully and it is simply impossible to gorge on these foods because your body tells you when you have eaten sufficient for your needs.

The fats in the New High Protein Diet are essential fats which you require for life: essential fatty acids such as omega-3 fatty acids (from fatty fish such as mackerel and salmon) and omega-6 fatty acids from seed oils (such as sesame seeds) or egg yolks.

As with the situation with protein in the diet, the *proportion* of fat increases in the diet rather than the *actual amount* of fat. Let us use the example given previously. If 100 grams of your current diet comprises 30 grams protein, 30 grams fat and 40 grams carbohydrate, the fat component is obviously 30%. When you remove the carbohydrates, you don't compensate by consuming much more protein or fats because, as we have already explained, protein and fats are much more satisfying to the appetite than carbohydrate so the same amount of fats – 30 grams – now assumes a 50% component of the 60-gram residual amount. In other words, the *same amount* of fat in the diet merely assumes a greater *proportion* of the diet.

Does this diet help to prevent diabetes?

There are basically two distinct forms of diabetes, aptly named Type 1 diabetes and Type 2 diabetes.

Type 1 diabetes usually occurs in early life and is caused by a deficiency of the hormone insulin, so doctors have to prescribe insulin injections to replace the missing insulin or the patient will die.

Type 2 diabetes is the commonest form of diabetes in the United Kingdom, comprising about 90% of diabetic patients. The features of Type 2 diabetes are almost the opposite of those in the Type 1 form of the condition, but the effects of raised blood sugar and serious complications affecting the eyes, kidneys and heart are the same in both forms. This usually occurs in later life and the patient actually produces too much insulin because the cells of the body are resistant to the effects of insulin. The more carbohydrates you consume, the more insulin you produce and the more your body becomes resistant to the effects of insulin so you have to produce even more insulin to have the same effect. So an increased consumption of refined carbohydrates causes massive increases in insulin production and a significantly increased risk of developing Type 2 diabetes. Reduce your intake of refined carbohydrates and your insulin production reduces dramatically, thereby reducing the risk of diabetes and its very serious complications, mainly eye disease, kidney disease and heart disease. The problem of diet is so severe in western society that doctors are now seeing the emergence of Type 2 diabetes – formerly a disease of the ageing population – in schoolchildren, almost certainly caused by a diet based on refined carbohydrates.

How does this diet affect my heart?

Two of the most important indicators of heart disease are blood levels of triglycerides and high-density-lipoprotein (HDL). High levels of triglycerides are harmful to the heart and high levels of HDL help protect the heart. Recent medical research comparing the effects of low-carbohydrate diets against low-calorie diets over periods of 6–12 months has shown that low-carb diets lowered the level of harmful triglycerides by 17% over one year, compared to unchanged levels in the low-calorie diet group, and increased the level of protective HDL by 11% over the same period, compared to less than 2% in the low-calorie group.

In simple terms, low-carb diets are not only much safer for the heart than low-calorie diets, the results suggest that low-carb diets actually *protect* the heart against thrombosis.

Chapter 4

How to Prepare Healthy Foods *Quickly*

The easiest way to enjoy healthy food *quickly* is to purchase food ready-cooked or ready to pop into the microwave. There are certainly many ready-cooked foods which are bursting with nutrients, such as chicken (breast, legs, thighs, wings), hams, salamis, beef, pork, continental sausages, mackerel, tuna, prawns . . . There are, however, even more 'fast' meals which are very unhealthy: pizzas, prepared 'microwave' meals (usually high in carbohydrates and low on nutrition), pies, oven-cooked or microwave chips, frozen pasta meals, quick-cook rice meals . . . The secret is to know which are healthy and which are not. As a simple guide, virtually *all* ready-cooked complete meals which are specifically designed for a low-calorie diet (usually frozen and microwavable) are high in carbohydrates and low in nutrients.

However it *is* easy to prepare fast nutritious and delicious meals from very healthy ingredients by following a few simple rules. The following advice on buying and cooking various foods will ensure you have a fast *and* healthy diet. Each section is divided into 'What to buy' and 'Cooking methods', which are the main problems for most people on any diet, healthy or otherwise.

Vegetables

What to buy

Buy fresh vegetables! If you want to be healthy and slim there is no alternative. Tinned and frozen vegetables have lost much of their natural flavour and in the case of tinned vegetables, usually contain added unhealthy ingredients such as salt and sugar.

But surely fresh vegetables take too much time in preparation for a fast food diet? Absolutely not! It's only root vegetables that take time in preparation and root vegetables are excluded from the weight loss phase of the diet. Peppers and mushrooms take minutes to slice and, as we have already discussed, most other vegetables can be purchased ready-washed and trimmed and ready to cook.

Individual fresh herbs are widely available from supermarkets, either packaged or growing in pots, so you can have a constant supply of fresh herbs from your kitchen if you wish. The cost is minimal, and a packet of fresh herb leaves will liven many meals (and the healthy antioxidant properties of herbs are unrivalled).

Cooking methods

There are many healthy ways of cooking vegetables. Different ways of cooking are appropriate to different foods. The best techniques of cooking vegetables to achieve both a quick and healthy result are:

- **Ready-prepared**

  Unlike other foods in this diet (such as meat, poultry and fish), vegetables cannot be purchased *ready-cooked* but they can be purchased *ready-prepared*, often pre-packaged for instant use. Carrots, broccoli, French beans, mangetout, sugar snap peas, cauliflower and beansprouts are just some of the myriad vegetables which can be purchased from supermarkets ready for instant use, either chopped or sliced, or topped and tailed. If you intend cooking a stir-fry meal, you can even purchase the appropriate mixture of pre-packed chopped vegetables for the individual type of meal. So there really is no reason why you cannot enjoy fresh vegetables of the highest nutritional value, even if you have no time for preparation. Stir-fried vegetables cook quickly, retaining most of their essential nutrients. With a prepared sauce and thin stir-fried strips of meat or poultry – or even shellfish – the entire meal can be prepared *and cooked* in less than 10 minutes, which is probably faster than a microwaved 'TV dinner' takes to cook, and infinitely healthier and more nutritious. Nutrients leach out of vegetables from the moment they are chopped, so the prepared variety are not quite as nutritious as fresh vegetables chopped immediately before use. However, some of us do not have the time in the evening to chop vegetables so pre-packaged fresh vegetables are the perfect solution to providing an instant source of the many essential vitamins, minerals and antioxidants which can only be obtained from this source.

Before leaving this subject, it would be useful to add a comment on the other forms of pre-packaged vegetables: tinned and frozen. Tinned vegetables have lost much of their intrinsic nutritional value, as the vegetables have been chopped and prepared for a relatively long period. And, in our experience, tinned vegetables are virtually tasteless! So there is really no necessity to resort to the tin-opener even if you don't have time to prepare fresh vegetables on a daily basis; the secret of successful dieting, once again, lies in *planning and shopping*.

Frozen vegetables are said to maintain their nutritional levels and are certainly useful for those with a very busy lifestyle, but, once again, in our experience frozen vegetables have a very mediocre taste compared to their fresh counterparts. With just a little forethought and planning you can use fresh pre-packaged vegetables in your meals to major benefit both in terms of taste and healthy nutrition. The purpose of eating is enjoyment, taste and health, all of which are integrally and inextricably related. Vegetables, although very healthy, can be prepared in various ways to be either delicious or basically unattractive; there is a world of difference between boiled cabbage and stir-fried vegetables in oyster sauce! Freshly prepared vegetables in packages are now widely available in many different combinations from supermarkets. They can be cooked rapidly, by either stir-frying or by microwave with various prepared sauces to produce a delicious meal in minutes, so there really is no need for the less nutritious option of tinned vegetables or the less tasty option of frozen vegetables.

Delicious salads are even easier! Most major supermarkets have an extensive range of prepared packaged salads, from baby spinach leaves, watercress and rocket, to various mixtures of different salad leaves. These form the perfect accompaniment to a main dish, such as meat, poultry or fish and provide a delicious and healthy meal with effectively negligible preparation time.

- **Stir-frying**
Stir-fried vegetables cook in a few minutes and retain most of their natural nutrition. The vegetables have to be sliced (or chopped) thinly for rapid cooking.

- **Steaming**
Steaming is a very healthy method of cooking as the vegetables lose virtually none of their nutrients and effectively cook themselves with very little attention required from the cook! The vegetables do not need to be sliced as thinly as in stir-frying for this method.

- **Microwaving**
  Cooking vegetables in the microwave is quick and healthy with most of the nutrients being retained. Once again, the vegetables cook themselves; ideal for the busy cook.

The only method of cooking vegetables to be avoided if possible is **boiling**. Boiling vegetables in water is time-consuming and unhealthy. Most of the nutrients leach out into the surrounding water and much of the taste and nutrition is lost.

Beef, Pork and Lamb

Beef, pork and lamb are prepared in comparable ways. The aim is to show you how easily you can cook fresh meats in virtually the same time it takes to cook a 'TV dinner'.

What to buy

With meats, you can either buy fresh and cook within a few days (or freeze for later) or buy frozen initially. The problem with buying frozen meat is that you have to remember to defrost it before use, so it's not that suitable for really fast suppers. Even defrosting meat by microwave is time-consuming and the aim of this diet is to be as user-friendly as possible. An alternative solution is to freeze some meat but keep most actually in the fridge. Most supermarket meats are pre-packaged and have a sell-by date several days in advance, so you can have instant access to fresh meats for many of the recipes in the book simply by keeping the meats in the fridge within their sell-by date.

Cooking methods

• Ready-cooked

Many meats can be purchased *ready cooked*, so there is no preparation or cooking time. Cold sliced meats are the obvious examples, however the choice extends much further: continental sausages, chorizo, salamis of various types, kabanos, hams, brackwurst, pastrami, pepperoni . . . Take a stroll through the cold meats section of your local delicatessen or supermarket and you will find an incredible selection which are virtually carbohydrate-free and which, therefore, are perfect for this diet.

• Frying

Frying meats (or stir-frying) in a moderate amount of extra-virgin olive oil is *not* unhealthy. On the contrary, extra-virgin olive oil is very healthy and the oils allow fat-soluble vitamins (A, D, E and K) to be absorbed from your foods. If there is no fat in your diet, you will inevitably become deficient in these essential nutrients because your body can't absorb the nutrients without some fat in the diet.

On the other hand, deep fat frying *is* unhealthy. The fat is raised to very high temperatures, which changes its constitution, and the duration of cooking can destroy the essential nutrients in the food.

So we can fry (or, even better, stir-fry) meat in a moderate amount of extra-virgin olive oil safely and healthily. When cooking, it is important to chop the meat to the appropriate size for the type of cooking. For example, minced beef fries more quickly than sirloin steak because it has a much larger surface area for the heat to penetrate the meat. So if you want to cook meat as quickly as possible, chop (or slice) the meat finely and it will be well-cooked in a matter of 3–4 minutes. Stir-fried meat should therefore be finely sliced. A steak will take twice as long to cook (obviously depending on personal preference) as it is much thicker.

- **Grilling**
Grilling is a very simple and quick method of cooking larger cuts of meat such as steaks and chops. A moderate steak will take 4–8 minutes (from rare to well-done), turning once, and requires very little preparation or supervision during cooking.

- **Baking**
Baking meat (in a casserole) takes a long time (usually up to 2 hours) so how can this method be included in a diet of this nature? Simply because the actual *preparation* time is relatively short: it only takes a few minutes to brown some pre-chopped beef, add gravy, tomatoes and herbs, and place in a pre-heated oven. Of course it takes 2 hours to cook, so it's not suitable for a weekday night, but the actual *preparation time* was less than 10 minutes. Providing you *plan* a little in advance, you can enjoy delicious, healthy casseroles which only actually take 10-15 minutes out of your day. In fact, casseroles are one of the fastest meals, because the meal cooks with little preparation and no supervision, leaving your time free until the meal is cooked.

- **Roasting**
Once again, roasting takes longer to cook *but a relatively short preparation time*. Obviously not convenient for a weekday night but eminently suitable for a delicious meal at the weekend with just a little forethought and preparation. It takes very little time (and effort) to place a joint of beef, lamb or pork in the oven and it is ready 1–2 hours later, and you have cold cuts for the next day for another delicious and nutritious meal.

- **Microwaving**
  Microwave cooking is perfect for many meat dishes.
  Preparation time is minimal, the meat cooks in a
  short time and the shrinkage is much less than in a
  conventional oven. And, most importantly, meat
  cooks in the microwave with very little supervision,
  so you can leave it to cook while you prepare the
  remainder of the meal.

Poultry

Poultry is probably the ultimate fast food which contains
all the essential amino acids we require for health, but
you have to learn to consider food in a totally different
way. Don't think of poultry as only roast chicken or
roast turkey. These are excellent meals and do not
require much preparation time, but they do require
considerable cooking time so they are only really
applicable to either those who have the convenience of
placing the chicken in the oven in the afternoon (which
excludes most of the population) or Sunday lunch, for
which these meals are obviously ideal.

What to buy
Poultry is definitely best bought fresh – although
chicken breast, wings, thighs and drumsticks can just
as easily be purchased freshly cooked! The cooked
variety are available immediately but, even with fresh
chicken, baking, stir-frying or microwaving are very
quick methods of cooking. Turkey is seldom available
ready-cooked (except sliced turkey breast) but fresh
turkey breast and drumsticks are widely available.
Turkey mince provides a delicious alternative to the
traditional minced beef with Bolognese sauce, or even
in burgers!

Cooking methods

• Ready-cooked

There is so much more to poultry than merely roast chicken. It can be purchased pre-cooked, as drumsticks, thighs, wings and breast. The pre-cooked varieties may be plain or have delicious sauces (such as chicken tikka, chinese or barbecue) which have very little carbohydrate content and are therefore perfect for a fast food low-carb diet. Chicken and turkey breast can also be purchased as sliced and cooked cold meats, again either plain or smoked. But always ensure pre-cooked chicken is purchased in sealed packages and are within the sell-by date. And always store in the fridge, and discard within 24 hours after opening. *Never* re-heat pre-cooked chicken.

• Stir-frying

Fresh poultry can also be cooked in a very short time, merely with a little preparation and forethought. Chicken breast can be chopped into cubes or strips and stir-fried in extra-virgin olive oil in just a few minutes. Add some pre-chopped vegetables, fresh ginger or garlic and a commercial sauce (oyster, chilli or hoisin, for example) and you have a delicious (and highly nutritious) meal in less than 15 minutes. This meal can actually require even less preparation time (if that seems possible) using thinly-sliced fresh turkey breast, which is available from most supermarkets. Sliced into thin strips, it requires no more than 2–3 minutes to stir-fry, add the vegetables and sauce, and the meal is ready in less than 10 minutes. For some reason, turkey breast is much cheaper than its chicken counterpart, so this is a very economical, nutritious and tasty alternative to the more traditional chicken.

- **Frying**

  Chicken or turkey breast can be shallow-fried in 2–3 tablespoons of extra-virgin olive oil. Turkey mince can be 'browned', then a delicious Bolognese sauce added or the mince can be formed into burgers and shallow-fried. Deep fat frying is not particularly healthy and there is really no reason to ever have to resort to this method of cooking.

- **Baking**

  Baking takes very little preparation time indeed: place the breast, drumsticks, wings or thighs on an oiled baking tray, and cook for 35–40 minutes in a pre-heated oven. Providing you remember to remove the chicken from the freezer in the morning (or have fresh chicken in the fridge, which is less likely for the average busy family in the average busy week), you can come home, place it in the oven, and continue with all the many tasks at the end of the day whilst the meal cooks itself.

- **Microwaving**

  Like meat, poultry cooks quickly and effortlessly in a microwave oven. Shrinkage is less and the poultry remains moist (if not overcooked).

- **Roasting**

  Finally, of course, there is always roasting the entire bird. Once again, the actual preparation time is minimal, the only delay is in the cooking time. However, providing you plan ahead, there is no reason not to enjoy roast chicken (or turkey or pheasant . . .) at the weekend. You simply plan your meal, put the bird in the oven and get on with your life while it cooks itself.

Fish and Shellfish

What to buy

Fish and shellfish always have more flavour when fresh, however the tinned varieties are just as nutritious and can be easily converted into delicious meals with the addition of sauces. Try to eat fish or shellfish *at least* twice a week, as they have many nutrients that are not as widely available in other foods. For example, 'oily fish' (mackerel, herring, sardines, salmon and tuna) are the best sources of essential omega-3 fatty acids in our diet and an excellent source of vitamin D (deficiency of which is the cause of 'brittle bones' or osteoporosis).

Cooking methods

- **Ready-cooked**

  There is an immense variety of pre-cooked fish and shellfish which are ready to eat and which provide all the essential amino acids for good health. Fish can be either pre-cooked and packaged (such as mackerel and smoked salmon) or tinned (such as salmon, tuna, sardines, mackerel, anchovies and herring). Similarly, shellfish are available either freshly cooked (prawns), tinned (crab, lobster, prawns), or even in sealed glass containers (cockles, winkles, whelks and mussels). All these can be quickly and easily combined with other prepared ingredients to create delicious – and very healthy – meals in less than 10 minutes. And pre-packaged fish and shellfish contain almost as many nutrients as the fresh variety, so they are very high in essential amino acids, vitamins, minerals and antioxidants.

  Frozen fish (haddock, cod and salmon) and frozen shellfish (prawns, tiger prawns, lobster and crab) can be defrosted and cooked in minutes (using a microwave oven) and are almost as instantly available as fresh produce. Once again, the fish and shellfish that have been frozen retain almost all their nutrition, so are still very healthy.

Of course, oysters are enjoyed raw with just a little lemon juice, and Japanese seafood meals are consumed raw; you can't really get much quicker (or more nutritious) than that!

• Stir-frying

Fish does not stir-fry well, as it tends to break up during cooking (especially very fresh fish). Calamari and shellfish (such as prawns and scallops), on the other hand, are very suitable for stir-frying as the meat is more compact.

• Frying

Fish are ideally suited for frying in a little extra-virgin olive oil (2–3 tablespoons) as they cook quickly and only require turning once, so the likelihood of 'breaking up' is lessened considerably.

• Baking

Once again, fish are ideally suited to baking as they will cook quickly (15–18 minutes) and require no supervision.

• Steaming

Both shellfish and fish are suitable for this very healthy form of cooking. All the nutrition is retained within the fish and shellfish, which cook quickly and without supervision.

• Grilling

Suitable for fish, but not shellfish as they tend to become very dry. Even fish can be very dry after this form of cooking, and as it requires supervision, grilling is not the most suitable form of cooking for the cook in a hurry!

- **Microwaving**
Microwave cooking is particularly suitable for fish and shellfish. Fresh fish fillets cook in three minutes and shellfish in even less time! The food retains moisture (and therefore texture) and all its essential nutrients.

Eggs

What to buy
If possible, large, fresh free-range eggs!

Cooking methods
Eggs are the ultimate fast food. They are packed full of nutrients such as essential amino acids, vitamins D, B_2, B_{12} and iodine. It is irrelevant which method of cooking is selected – providing they are not *overcooked*. Eggs can be poached, scrambled, baked or made into omelettes by the traditional methods which are reasonably quick, but have the disadvantage of requiring supervision during cooking and tedious washing of pans afterwards; or the eggs can be similarly cooked in the microwave oven, very quickly, without supervision and with minimal washing-up.

- Poached
- Boiled
- Scrambled
- Fried
- Baked
- Omelette
- Microwave

Chapter 5

Breakfast

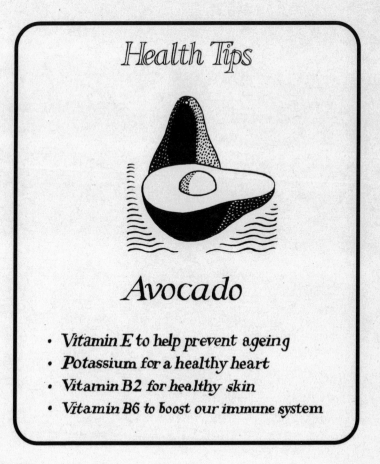

Health Tips

Avocado

- *Vitamin E to help prevent ageing*
- *Potassium for a healthy heart*
- *Vitamin B2 for healthy skin*
- *Vitamin B6 to boost our immune system*

Boiled eggs	85
Scrambled eggs	85–86
Omelette	87–88
Poached eggs	89–90
Fried eggs	90–91
Bacon and gammon	91–93
Toasted cheese	93–95
Kippers	96–97
Trout with coriander and lemon butter sauce	97–98
Whiting with herbs	98–99
Haddock with grilled Leerdammer	99–100
Sardines with herbs	100
Whiting with scrambled eggs and basil	100–101
Smoked haddock with poached eggs	101–102
Mushrooms with bacon	102–103
Tomatoes with mushrooms	103
Avocado on toast	104

Breakfast is essential for a successful diet! The single most important factor in preventing unnecessary (and disastrous) snacking during the day is ensuring that you are *never hungry*, which means starting the day with a healthy, and satisfying, breakfast. Of course, some people just can't face breakfast first thing in the morning and we will provide solutions to this common problem, but it is important to satisfy your morning appetite by 10 am or you will inevitably snack on the wrong types of food simply because you are hungry. Once again, it is important to repeat that a successful diet must be tailored to fit your lifestyle, not the other way around, or it is bound to fail. We will provide a dietary programme which can be adapted to virtually every lifestyle, no matter how hectic, but obviously you will have to follow some of the suggestions for your diet to succeed and one of the most important is that you must eat a satisfying meal before 10 am.

A healthy, nutritious and satisfying breakfast does not have to be time-consuming or expensive, but it obviously has to adhere to the simple principles of the diet, so:

- a maximum of one slice of wholemeal bread or toast (preferably none)
- no cereals
- no pastries/croissants
- no jams or marmalade
- no fruit juice (during the weight loss phase of the diet)

- only one piece of fruit per day (during the weight loss phase of the diet)

Having excluded the refined carbohydrates, the remaining possibilities are almost infinite. A *real* fast-food breakfast can be either:

- at home
- at a bistro
- take-away

Irrespective of where the breakfast is enjoyed, the principles of the diet remain the same.

Quick and healthy breakfast at home

Quick, nutritious and healthy breakfast, which is also very satisfying and guaranteed to comply with your weight-loss programme, does *not* need to take much time. It merely requires a little forward planning. The problem is that we are all in a hurry in the morning and this has been the basis of the success of the carbohydrate breakfast over the past 40 years. When you are rushing and need a quick burst of energy, what could be easier than a bowl of cereal and a slice of toast with marmalade? You get the energy you require from the sugar in the meal and you feel better, but within a couple of hours you begin to feel weak and irritable again (because your sugar levels have dropped) so you have a biscuit or pastry with a cup of coffee and you feel better for another hour or two. Then the same symptoms return and you literally *have* to eat again, often a hasty sandwich or ciabatta or bagel or fast-food pasta or pizza for lunch. And the carbohydrate cycle continues into the afternoon, almost inevitably culminating in an evening meal which is based on pasta, rice or pizza, or with some form of potatoes, such as chips.

Pause for a moment to consider how this type of diet is absolutely guaranteed to build fat *even if you are careful to count calories*. When you start the day with cereal and toast, you have a sudden rise in blood sugar levels which makes you feel better for a short time but this stimulates the hormone insulin to be produced which rapidly *lowers* your blood sugar so you feel irritable and weak a couple of hours later, and you simple have to eat again. Even worse, *the insulin converts the sugar to fat*, as that is one of the main functions of insulin. So by following a diet based on refined carbohydrates, it is a self-sustaining process which virtually guarantees becoming fat. The only way in which you can prevent fat production on a carbohydrate-based diet is by extreme exercise and as very few adults run daily marathons this is not a viable alternative!

Let us look at the medical effects of a diet *without* refined carbohydrates. Breakfast on scrambled eggs (with chopped chives and basil) and tomatoes, a take-away lunch of a toasted open-sandwich piled with ham and Emmental cheese and dinner consisting of sliced beef in oyster sauce with stir-fried vegetables, and all in *virtually unlimited quantities*. A grand total of 35 grams of carbohydrate for the day, virtually no significant stimulation of the insulin response, so no conversion of the calories to fat! The breakfast of scrambled eggs will slow the digestion and satisfy hunger for several hours. No lowering of blood sugar, so no irritability or weakness mid-morning. Lunch can be as large or as small as you wish, providing you severely restrict the refined carbohydrates. So you *can* have an *open* sandwich (with only one slice of bread), and eat virtually as much low-carb (or no-carb) filling as you want, and you will still lose weight quickly and easily.

Some celebrities follow these guidelines to extreme levels: we were in a television hospitality room after recording a programme recently with a well-known television personality who was famous for her slim appearance. She proceeded to eat most of the sandwiches, consuming the fillings and discarding the bread! We would not advocate this extreme approach but, providing you limit your bread intake to a maximum of one slice per day, you will keep the carbs down and you will lose weight. As an added bonus, you will be becoming healthier by consuming nutrients which are essential for the efficient functioning of the body, so by dieting to lose weight you will feel much better, and will be healthier – and all without willpower or hunger, just a sensible approach to healthy eating!

Let us explain how easy it is to overcome the time problem, even for the busiest working mother with young children to prepare for school before leaving for work. This is probably the worst case scenario; the difficulties for anyone else *have* to be less than this! There are many quick-and-easy breakfasts which are both delicious and nutritious. The secret is having the necessary ingredients available, and preparation. And the other secret is a microwave oven. While it is not essential to own a microwave oven, they are relatively inexpensive at present and they allow healthy food to be cooked in minutes *whilst you can be busy with some of the other essential tasks in the morning.* A microwave oven is the perfect breakfast cooker for the busy person.

For example, poached eggs can be cooked in the microwave in 1½ minutes, while you are busy with some other task, as can scrambled eggs. Mixed with some chopped fresh herbs, possibly on a slice of wholemeal toast with chopped tomatoes and the entire exercise can take less than five minutes! Or possibly grill ham, bacon or gammon steak; although these can also be cooked in a microwave oven without supervision. Grilled or fried mushrooms on wholemeal toast; tinned tomatoes with fresh or dried herbs on a slice of wholemeal toast (the toast is optional); Continental-style breakfast with a selection of ham, cheeses, sliced meats (salami, chorizo, pastrami, ham, chicken or turkey) with a single piece of fruit and either a slice of wholemeal toast or a toasted bagel can all be ready in less than 5 minutes. Amazingly, a full cooked breakfast, with a selection of bacon, eggs, sausages, tomatoes and mushrooms can also be cooked in a microwave oven in less than 5 minutes!

The secret is having the appropriate healthy foods available. And these foods, as well as increasing your health and ensuring a successful diet, will actually save you money as they satisfy hunger for hours, preventing the low blood sugar mid-morning which occurs with a carbohydrate-based diet – so you won't have to buy expensive pastries, croissants or bagels mid-morning!

Continental breakfast

Without doubt, the 'fastest' breakfast is a Continental style – without the pastries, croissants and jams! Be adventurous. Many delicious foods are low-carb – or no-carb – and ideal for this style of breakfast. Here are a selection of foods which can be included safely and healthily in a low-carb diet but check your supermarket or delicatessen as there are many more which fit the low-carb criteria perfectly.

Cheeses

Almost all cheeses have virtually no carbohydrates, so they are perfect for inclusion in the diet and the immense variety of different cheeses allows for an almost infinite variation on the Continental breakfast. And cheese has the economic advantage that it can be purchased in small quantities, so you could buy small amounts of seven different cheeses for each day of the week. You don't need much cheese at breakfast for it to be completely satisfying; in fact, as cheese is very 'filling', not only will it satisfy your appetite at breakfast, it slows the digestion which means that you are not hungry throughout the morning.

Try different cheeses, especially those you have never previously tasted. Even relatively expensive cheeses are inexpensive when purchased in small quantities, which is all you will need. Don't restrict yourself to Cheddar, search your delicatessen (or supermarket) for as wide a variety as you can. Unless you are particularly partial to strong cheese, such as Stilton or Roquefort, milder cheeses are more appropriate at breakfast. The following cheeses blend well with the other diverse flavours of this breakfast style and do not overpower the meal. Enjoying cheeses is like a world tour of instant 'fast' food:

- Edam, Gouda and Leerdammer from Holland.
- Emmental and Gruyere from Switzerland.
- Jarlsberg from Norway.
- Brie, Camembert, Port Salut and St Nectaire from France.
- Taleggio, Fontina, Bocconcini, mozzarella and pecorino from Italy.
- Kefalotyri, Halloumi and feta from Greece.

And this is only the tip of the iceberg; the potential choices are literally endless.

Tomatoes and avocados

Tomatoes (especially plum tomatoes) and avocados are perfect additions to any breakfast – cooked or raw – for both taste and nutritional value. Tomatoes are an important source of vitamin A and the antioxidant 'lycopene', and avocados are a rich source of another antioxidant, vitamin E. As avocados have a natural fat content, they also slow the digestion allowing slower absorption of food and preventing hunger for longer.

Hams

In addition to providing an excellent source of all our essential amino acids, pork provides a particularly rich source of vitamin B_1 so it should be included in your diet if possible.

There are cooked hams available to suit every possible individual taste; the following provides a brief indication of the multitude of different hams which can be incorporated into this diet:

- Leg ham, champagne ham, honey ham, smoked ham and shaved ham from the United Kingdom.
- Parma ham and pancetta from Italy.
- Kasseler, Rohschinken, Lachschinken and Black Forest ham from Germany.

Continental sausages

Continental sausages are pre-cooked and ready to enjoy. Most are pure meats with added herbs and spices, so they are virtually carbohydrate-free, but be careful of any cheaper varieties as they may have 'hidden' carbohydrates as fillers to replace the meat. They taste delicious, and can be enjoyed – virtually without restriction – on a low-carb diet. Many varieties contain a combination of different meats, however this has no adverse effects on the diet, as the carbohydrate content of *all* meat is negligible. Your delicatessan or supermarket will have an extensive variety available and some excellent examples you may wish to include in your diet are:

- Frankfurters, from Germany – either pure pork with spices, or pork and beef.

- Luciana, from Italy – pure pork with herbs.
- Bockwurst, from Germany – smoked beef and pork.
- Salsicces, from Italy – pork and pancetta with herbs, spices and garlic.
- Strassburg, from Germany – beef and pork with coriander and pepper.
- Kabanas, from Poland – spicy pork.
- Brockwurst, from Germany – beef and pork with spices.
- Provencal, from France – spicy pork and beef with garlic.
- Schauessen, from Germany – pork and beef.

Unfortunately some (not all) British sausages contain a significant amount of carbohydrate. Read the label on the packaging to ensure it is pure meat, or at least low in carbohydrate content, and you will be safe to include them in your healthy low-carb diet.

Salami
Salami has virtually no carbohydrate content and tastes delicious, so it can be included – virtually without restriction – in a healthy low-carb diet. Don't worry about the calories; providing you keep the carbs to low levels (less than 40–60 grams per day), the calories cannot be deposited as fat and are of no relevance to your diet! Once again, you won't overindulge as salami naturally satisfies your appetite. One of the delightful qualities of salami – as with most prepared meats – is the tremendous variety available, reflecting the diversity of different recipes in different countries. Most salamis consist of pork and/or beef. A brief selection of some available, which are low-carb and therefore eminently suitable to be included in this diet are:

- Chorizo from Spain – pork with spices.
- Pepperoni – with red pepper seasoning.

- Milano – spicy salami.
- Florentino – mild spicy salami.
- Siciliano – hot and salty.
- Napoli – pork and beef with pepper.
- Calabrese – hot and spicy with added chillies.
- Felinetti – mild salami with pepper and garlic.
- Contadino – spicy with whole peppercorns.
- Cresponi – mild and dense.
- Toscana – slightly sweet.
- Casalinga – hot with garlic and spices.
- Cayenne – very hot with Cayenne pepper.
- Mettwurst – made with pork.
- Gyulai – smoked salami with red pepper.
- Cacciatore – with garlic and spices.
- Csabai – spicy with paprika and peppercorns.

These, and many more, are available in delicatessens, although there is an equally impressive array available in supermarkets. Almost all salami can be included in this diet but remember to always **read the label** on pre-packaged food, as sometimes a manufacturer has added sugar or carbohydrate. Pure salami is virtually carbohydrate-free.

Beef
All forms of beef are suitable for this diet, as beef is virtually carbohydrate-free.

- Pastrami – cured and spiced beef, often rubbed with chilli and peppercorns.
- Salt beef – cured brisket of beef.
- Smoked beef – cured and smoked beef.

Poultry
Poultry, like beef, is virtually carbohydrate-free, so it is ideal for inclusion in this delicious diet. For a fast-food breakfast, you can either cook chicken/turkey breast (or drumsticks) the previous evening (see pages 62–64),

81

or purchase it ready-cooked from the supermarket; the choice available, once again, is huge, from chicken breast, drumsticks, thighs and wings. The ready-cooked chicken may have added sauce for extra flavour (such as barbecue, tikka or Chinese), so check the label to make sure that there is not too much sugar in the sauce as this can ruin the diet. Most sauces in pre-packed chicken only add 1–2 grams of carbohydrate per 100 grams, so they are of little significance.

Eggs

Eggs are perfect for the diet (whether boiled, poached, fried, scrambled or as an omelette) as they provide all essential amino acids, many vitamins (especially vitamin B_{12}) and minerals, and are virtually carbohydrate-free. To include eggs in a Continental-style breakfast, simply hard-boil a large free-range egg for about 6 minutes whilst you are busy preparing the rest of the breakfast and it will be ready by the time you are ready to eat.

Fish

Don't forget fish for breakfast! Until comparatively recently, fish was a breakfast staple. And it was a relatively inexpensive meal: kippers and oysters were the staple diet of the poor, not the rich! Whilst we will address the subject of cooked fish for breakfast a little later in the chapter, *pre*-cooked fish can easily – and very healthily – be included in a Continental-style breakfast. Pre-cooked mackerel, or smoked mackerel, is widely available in supermarkets; sardines, or a little smoked salmon, are delicious accompaniments to a Continental breakfast. And each of these fish is relatively inexpensive: mackerel and sardines (fresh or tinned) are among the cheapest of fish and although smoked salmon seems expensive, you can only consume a little at a time because it has a very 'rich' taste (especially if combined with mayonnaise), so

100 grams would be sufficient for 3 breakfast meals. When you consider the cost this way, smoked salmon is really quite economical. All three fish provide excellent nutrition as they are rich sources of omega 3 essential fats, vitamin D and calcium.

Fruit

Fruit is not 'forbidden' on the diet, merely severely restricted in the weight loss phase, as it contains a relatively high proportion of natural sugars. You can have one piece of fruit for breakfast if you wish, but restrict it to one of the following:

- Apple – 10 grams of carbohydrate
- Apricot – 7 grams of carbohydrate
- Blackberries (100 grams) – 12 grams of carbohydrate
- Blueberries (100 grams) – 13 grams of carbohydrate
- Cherries (100 grams) – 12 grams of carbohydrate
- Gooseberries (100 grams) – 13 grams of carbohydrate
- Grapefruit (100 grams) – 10 grams of carbohydrate
- Grapes (100 grams) – black: 15 grams of carbohydrate
  green: 12 grams of carbohydrate
- Kiwi fruit – 7 grams of carbohydrate
- Lemon – 3 grams of carbohydrate
- Lime – 1 gram of carbohydrate
- Manderine – 4 grams of carbohydrate
- Melon – honeydew melon (100 grams): 6 grams of carbohydrate
  rock melon (100 grams): 5 grams of carbohydrate
  watermelon (100 grams): 5 grams of carbohydrate
- Nectarine – 7 grams of carbohydrate
- Orange – 10 grams of carbohydrate

- Passion fruit – 3 grams of carbohydrate
- Peach – 8 grams of carbohydrate
- Pear – 16 grams of carbohydrate
- Pineapple (100 grams) – 8 grams of carbohydrate
- Plum – 8 grams of carbohydrate
- Raspberries (100 grams) – 5 grams of carbohydrate
- Rhubarb (100 grams) – 1 gram of carbohydrate
- Strawberries (100 grams) – 6 grams of carbohydrate
- Tangerine – 7 grams of carbohydrate

As you can see, fruit *can* be included in the diet in moderation providing you restrict the amount. As the average slice of bread contains about 17 grams of carbohydrate, you would be much better advised to include some fruit in your daily 40–60 grams of carbohydrate *rather than bread*, which has very little nutritional value. The carbohydrate content of each *average* piece of fruit is provided to ensure that you do not exceed your carbohydrate limit for the day. Bananas and mangoes are fruits which are high in carbohydrates and therefore *definitely* to be avoided. Fruit is one of the few items included in the diet for which you *must* measure the amount you consume, simply because it is relatively high in carbohydrate content.

Cooked breakfast

Cooked breakfast is usually not considered appropriate or feasible during the working week as it takes too long to prepare, but this need not be the case. Cooked in the microwave oven it takes only a few minutes. The food cooks *without supervision*, so the time element is negligible and the nutritional benefits over the standard, high-carb 'cereal and toast' are immense.

Boiled eggs

Boiled eggs are the only method of cooking eggs in which the traditional method is probably superior to microwave cooking because the microwave technique requires a dedicated egg-boiler dish. Even so, we have not described a microwave method for boiling eggs.

For 2
2 large (preferably free-range eggs)

Traditional method

- Place 2 large eggs in warm water, bring to the boil, then reduce the heat to a gentle boil. Excessive boiling will spoil the flavour and often causes the eggs to crack. The length of time depends on how you prefer your boiled eggs: with large eggs, between 3 minutes for soft-boiled to 8 minutes for hard-boiled.

You can obviously have the boiled eggs alone (or with a single slice of wholemeal toast), or hard boil the eggs and add to a Continental-style breakfast (see pages 77 and 82).

CARBOHYDRATE CONTENT PER SERVING: NEGLIGIBLE (WITHOUT TOAST); 17 GRAMS (WITH TOAST)

Scrambled eggs

Scrambled eggs are ideally suited to microwave cooking. Traditional methods are labour-intensive as the eggs need to be constantly supervised initially, then stirred. And washing a pan in which scrambled eggs have been cooked is definitely labour-intensive!

Scrambled eggs cooked in a microwave is exactly the opposite. The eggs cook without supervision to perfection and there is only a single bowl to clean afterwards. We have provided both methods, but we would not advocate a traditional method as a realistic option on a hectic weekday morning.

For 2

   3 large eggs (preferably free-range)
   2 tbsp full-cream milk
   freshly ground black pepper
   25 grams butter

By microwave

- Add the beaten eggs to a microwave-safe bowl and place in the centre of the microwave oven. Set on 'high' and cook for one minute.
- Remove the bowl from microwave, and stir the mixture, bringing the edges to the centre.
- Return to microwave and cook on 'high' for another minute, and repeat.
- Repeat the process for another minute or until the mixture just begins to set.

Traditional method

- Break the eggs in a mixing bowl.
- Add the milk and a little freshly ground black pepper, and beat gently with a fork to an even consistency.
- Melt the butter in a small pan over a low heat, and add the eggs.
- Stir constantly, moving the edges to the middle with a circular motion, for about 2–3 minutes.
- Remove from heat when the eggs are no longer runny (before the eggs have set) to allow the heat of the pan to gently finish the cooking, and serve.

Scrambled eggs are delicious alone but even better with a tasty accompaniment. The possibilities are virtually infinite: here are some suggestions. These suggestions are not intended to be mutually exclusive and you can add different combinations too.

- 2 spring onions, finely chopped
- 1 tbsp chopped fresh basil

- 50 grams grated Leerdammer cheese (or any other cheese according to your preference)
- 50 grams smoked salmon, finely chopped
- 1 tbsp chopped fresh chives
- 1 tsp balsamic vinegar
- 50 grams chopped smoked mackerel
- 1 tbsp chopped fresh coriander
- 50 grams smoked ham, finely chopped
- 25 grams button mushrooms, sliced and sautéed in 30 grams butter
- 25 grams chorizo sausage, finely diced
- 1 medium plum tomato on-the-vine, deseeded and finely diced
- 25 grams pre-cooked prawns
- 1 tsp Worcestershire sauce with 50 grams chopped, fresh flat-leaf parsley

CARBOHYDRATE CONTENT PER SERVING: 2–3 GRAMS, DEPENDING ON ADDED INGREDIENTS

Omelette

For 2
3 large eggs (preferably free-range)
freshly ground black pepper
2 tbsp full-cream milk
25 grams butter

Omelettes can be cooked quite quickly by the conventional method but it does require supervision. However, by microwave you simply place the egg mixture in the oven and enjoy it 3 minutes later!

By microwave
- Whisk the eggs, seasoning and milk with a fork to an even consistency.
- Pour half of the mixture into each side of the microwave omelette maker.

- Do not close the omelette maker. Place in the microwave cooker and cook on 'high' for 1 minute.
- Lift the edges of the omelette to allow the uncooked egg mixture to run under the cooked portion.
- Return the open omelette maker to the microwave oven and cook on 'high' for a further minute.
- Add the desired filling, then close the omelette maker, return to the microwave oven and cook on 'high' for a final 30 seconds.
- Slide the cooked omelette onto a warm plate.

Traditional method

- Whisk the eggs, seasoning and milk with a fork to an even consistency.
- Melt the butter in an omelette pan, tilting the pan to ensure an even coating of butter. When the butter is hot add the egg mixture.
- Stir the mixture with a fork until the omelette just begins to set.
- Add the filling.
- Cook the omelette for about another minute, then, using a palette knife, gently lift one edge of the omelette, fold one half over the other and slide the omelette onto a plate.

Omelettes are a perfect accompaniment to any low-carb diet as they are so versatile. As you now appreciate, an omelette can be adapted for breakfast even in the most hectic household, and, although delicious in itself, the potential range of healthy, low-carb fillings are virtually infinite. Here are a few suggestions, however you probably have your own favourites. As all the fillings are very low in carbohydrates, you can vary the quantities and still keep to the diet.

- 50 grams button mushrooms, sliced and lightly sautéed

- 1 tbsp chopped fresh basil and spring onion, finely diced
- 3 slices pre-cooked turkey breast, finely diced, with 1 tsp of cranberry sauce
- 50 grams grated Roquefort cheese and 1 tbsp chopped fresh chives
- 50 grams cooked prawns
- ½ small Hass avocado (peeled and stone removed), diced with 1 medium plum tomato, diced
- 50 grams smoked salmon, thinly sliced
- 50 grams sliced Parma ham with 1 tsp Dijon mustard
- 4 thin slices of mozzarella cheese and 1 tsp balsamic vinegar
- 2 shallots (peeled and diced) with 1 garlic clove (peeled and diced), sautéed in 50 grams butter

CARBOHYDRATE CONTENT PER SERVING: 2–3 GRAMS
(DEPENDING ON ADDED INGREDIENTS)

Poached eggs

For 2
2 large preferably free-range eggs
½ tsp grated nutmeg or paprika
freshly ground black pepper

Poached eggs are an excellent dish on a low-carb diet. They contain virtually no carbohydrate, taste delicious and slow the digestion, satisfying the appetite for hours and removing the desire to 'snack' during the morning. But, the conventional method of poaching eggs is definitely time-consuming; once again, poaching eggs by microwave is quick and easy. In fact, it's almost as quick as cereal and toast – and infinitely healthier!

By microwave
- Break each egg individually into the plastic cups specially designed for poaching eggs in the microwave.

- Pierce the tops of the yolks 4–5 times with a sharp knife, add a teaspoon of cold water, and close the top of the cup to seal.
- Cook on medium (be careful, on 'high' it will explode!) for about 1½ minutes (depending on the power of the microwave), then allow to stand for another minute before serving.
- Serve on a slice of buttered wholemeal toast, sprinkle over a little grated nutmeg or paprika and season to taste with freshly ground black pepper.

Traditional method

- Heat the water to boiling point in a shallow pan, then reduce the heat to a gentle simmer.
- Break each egg individually into a cup, then slide the eggs gently into the boiling water.
- Cook for approximately 3–4 minutes, removing the eggs from the water with a perforated spoon when the yolk is evenly coated with a white film and the white has cooked.
- Serve on a slice of buttered wholemeal toast, sprinkle over a little grated nutmeg or paprika and season to taste with freshly ground black pepper.

CARBOHYDRATE CONTENT PER SERVING: NEGLIGIBLE
(WITHOUT TOAST); 17 GRAMS (WITH TOAST)

Fried eggs

Eggs can be 'fried' in a microwave, but to obtain the desired appearance and effect involves heating a special tray in a conventional oven for a few minutes, then cooking the eggs (and bacon/tomatoes/mushrooms) on the hot tray in the microwave. As this probably involves more effort than the conventional method of cooking fried eggs, the traditional technique is probably superior.

And, of course, because eggs contain very little

carbohydrate, you will continue to lose weight even though the eggs are fried because the calories are not converted to fat unless there is carbohydrate to stimulate the production of insulin, which in turn stimulates the body to deposit calories as body fat.

For 2
4 tbsp extra-virgin olive oil
2 large preferably free-range eggs
4 rashers bacon (optional)

Traditional method

- Pour about 4 tablespoons extra-virgin olive oil into the (preferably non-stick) frying pan.
- Heat the oil until it is hot but not burning, and gently crack the eggs into the pan. The eggs are then cooked to taste, either sunny-side up, over-easy (turning the eggs), or simply by basting the hot oil over the egg with a spatula. Once again, the duration of cooking is a matter of personal preference, depending upon how well you like your eggs cooked.
- When cooked to taste, remove the eggs with a perforated spatula. Serve either alone or with a combination of grilled bacon, gammon, mushrooms or tomatoes.

CARBOHYDRATE CONTENT PER SERVING: NEGLIGIBLE

Bacon and gammon

Bacon and gammon are ideal for breakfast as they are quickly cooked, slow the digestion (so your appetite is satisfied for longer), are very nutritious (providing all the essential amino acids) and taste delicious. Frying is not particularly appropriate for a quick breakfast as it is time-consuming and requires constant supervision.

Grilling is easier, but by far the fastest and most convenient method in the morning is by microwave, where the bacon is cooked within 3 minutes with no supervision. Specially designed plastic microwave bacon cookers can be purchased inexpensively; the best types have a ribbed tray on the base to allow even cooking and a cover to prevent 'spitting' of the bacon during cooking.

For 2
6 rashers bacon

By microwave

- Lay the bacon rashers evenly in a single layer on the ribbed base of the tray.
- Replace the cover and place the plastic container in the microwave oven.
- Cook on 'high' for about 3 minutes, turning the bacon once after 1½ minutes.
- Serve immediately.

Grilled

- Heat the grill.
- Place the rashers of bacon on a grill tray and slide it into the oven, no closer than 8–10cm from the grill.
- Cook under a hot grill for 2 minutes per side, turning once.
- Serve immediately.

CARBOHYDRATE CONTENT PER SERVING: NEGLIGIBLE

Bacon can be replaced by a single gammon steak which will easily provide breakfast for two and the bacon (or gammon) can be enjoyed with grilled tomatoes or mushrooms or even poached eggs. Cooked in the microwave oven, poached eggs take less than 2 minutes, so the entire time necessary to prepare bacon and poached eggs is less than 5 minutes! And as there is no need for supervision in this type of cooking, you can be busy with other tasks while your meal is cooking, so the actual time it takes to cook the meal is the time taken to place the bacon and eggs in the cooker as the meal cooks itself.

The comparison which always has to be made is with cereal and toast – probably the commonest breakfast in busy households – not on the basis of taste but rather because it is so quick and convenient. By cooking in a microwave oven, you can literally cook bacon and eggs in almost the same time it takes to pour the cereal and milk and make the toast. It tastes delicious and you have the perfect nutritious, low-carb start to the day.

Cheese
Cheese is perfect for breakfast, either 'cold' in Continental-style breakfast or toasted. With all the essential amino acids for health and an excellent source of vitamin D, cheese is a highly nutritious food which should be included in any healthy diet (unless, of course, you don't like cheese). It contains virtually no carbohydrate and is therefore perfectly suited to a low-carb diet. The fat in cheeses slows the absorption of food and satisfies appetite, if you have it at breakfast, so you will not be hungry again until lunch.

Toasted cheese

Toasted cheese is a delicious breakfast; the only disadvantage is that you need bread, but a single slice of wholemeal toast will only add 15–17 grams of carbohydrate to your diet. Try different cheeses or even mix cheeses for added variety.

For 2
  2 slices wholemeal bread
  cheese, thinly sliced
  5–6 drops Worcestershire sauce
  freshly ground black pepper

Traditional method

- Lightly toast one side of a slice of wholemeal bread, then remove from the grill.
- Butter the other side.
- Lay slices of cheese on the non-toasted side, drizzle over a few drops of Worcestershire sauce and return to the grill until the cheese has melted.
- Season with freshly ground black pepper, then serve alone, or with a little pickle.

Almost all cheeses taste delicious toasted, simply because the meal essentially consists of cheese, each of which has a completely unique flavour. Try the following for a spectrum of the flavours of different cheeses:

- Mozzarella
- Fontini
- Edam
- Tallegio
- Port Salut
- Emmental
- Roquefort
- Gouda
- Jarlsberg
- Red Leicester
- Kefalotyri
- Brie
- Gruyere
- Bocconcini
- Leerdammer

- Feta
- Camembert
- Parmesan

While toasted cheese is delicious alone, there are an infinite array of potential accompaniments which create totally new and delicious meals in seconds:

- 1 tbsp chopped fresh chives
- 1 slice salami (of choice) with 1 tsp Dijon mustard
- dash of Balsamic vinegar
- 1 slice cooked turkey breast, diced
- 1 tbsp chopped fresh basil and flat-leaf parsley
- 1 slice pastrami with diced spring onion
- 1 tbsp chopped fresh chives and basil
- honey ham, finely diced, with 1 tsp of wholegrain mustard
- 1 medium plum tomato-on-the-vine, sliced, with 1 tbsp chopped fresh oregano
- finely diced smoked salmon

CARBOHYDRATE CONTENT PER SERVING: 17–20 GRAMS
(INCLUDING THE TOAST)

Fish

Fish is a delicious, healthy food which is suitable for every meal from light breakfast to dinner. Obviously, as with all foods, different fish and different methods of cooking are appropriate for different times of day; for example, cod mornay would not be easily prepared – or even suitable – as a breakfast dish. On the other hand, smoked haddock with herbs is a delicious breakfast meal.

Breakfast should be healthy and light but totally satisfying, and fish fit these requirements perfectly. With essential fatty acids, all essential amino acids, vitamins and minerals, there really is no healthier start to the day and the cooking time is minimal when you know the quick methods of cooking.

Kippers

Kippers, or smoked herring, can be cooked quickly in many ways: grilled, poached, fried or by microwave. Simply choose the method that you prefer, and if you don't like bones buy kipper fillets instead of whole kippers.

For 1
1 kipper
1 tbsp extra-virgin olive oil
60 grams of butter
1 plum tomato, diced
1 tbsp chopped fresh basil
freshly ground black pepper
lemon wedge (optional)

By microwave

- Place the kipper in a shallow microwave-safe dish, brush with extra-virgin olive oil and cover.
- Cook on high for 2 minutes, then allow to stand for 3–4 minutes.
- Transfer the kipper to a warm plate and season to taste.
- Sprinkle over the basil and lemon juice and serve with chopped tomato.

Grilled

- Heat the grill.
- Remove the head and tail then place the kippers on a grill tray, skin side uppermost. Brush with extra-virgin olive oil and grill under a hot grill (no closer than 8 cm from the grill) for 1–2 minutes.
- Turn over the kipper and grill for a further 3–4 minutes.
- Season to taste, sprinkle over the basil and lemon juice.
- Serve with chopped tomato.

Fried
- Heat the butter in a shallow frying pan, add the kipper and cook for 2 minutes on each side.
- Season to taste, sprinkle over the basil and lemon juice.
- Serve with chopped tomato.

Poached (or 'jugged')
- Remove the head, then place the kipper in a jug filled with boiling water, cover and leave for 4–5 minutes.
- Drain, season to taste, sprinkle over the basil and lemon juice.
- Serve with chopped tomato.

CARBOHYDRATE CONTENT PER SERVING: 3 GRAMS

Trout with coriander and lemon butter sauce

Few people would consider trout for breakfast but that is only because it is not a recognised breakfast meal. In fact, trout fits the criteria for breakfast perfectly: a light nutritious meal which tastes delicious and can be cooked very quickly.

For 2
2 medium trout fillets
60 grams butter
1 tbsp chopped fresh coriander leaves
juice of a freshly squeezed lemon
1 tsp chopped fresh chives
freshly ground black pepper

By microwave
By far the easiest method of cooking trout in the morning is by microwave. Quicker and easier, with less fuss and less washing up!

- Lay the fillets in a shallow microwave-safe dish and cover.
- Cook on 'high' for 2 minutes, then allow to stand for 1 minute.

At the same time

- Heat the butter in a small saucepan until melted, then stir in the coriander leaves and lemon juice.
- To serve the trout, drizzle over the coriander and lemon butter sauce, garnish with chopped chives and season to taste.

Pan fried
- Heat the butter in the pan and sauté the trout fillets for about 1–1½ minutes per side, turning carefully once with a fish slice.
- Serve the fillets onto warm plates.
- Add the coriander to the butter in the pan, stir in the lemon juice and heat gently for a few seconds.
- Pour the sauce over the fish and season to taste.
- Garnish with chopped chives.

CARBOHYDRATE CONTENT PER SERVING: 1 GRAM

Whiting with herbs

Another fish which is not a recognised breakfast option but this fish, again, satisfies all the essential criteria for a healthy start to the day. Whiting are small fillets which can therefore be purchased in small quantities, allowing for variety at breakfast which is an essential part of the enjoyment of food. The fillets are light and tasty, and cook in minutes in the microwave without supervision. With some fresh herbs you have the perfect meal. Baking takes a little more time in preparation, but similarly requires no supervision during cooking.

For 2
4 small whiting fillets
100 ml full-cream milk
1 tbsp chopped fresh basil
1 tbsp chopped fresh dill
freshly ground black pepper

By microwave

- Place the whiting fillets in a microwave-safe dish and cover.
- Cook on high for 2 minutes.
- Allow to stand for 1 minute, then serve immediately garnished with fresh basil and dill.

Baking

- Place the whiting fillets in an oven-safe dish, add the full-cream milk and chopped fresh herbs.
- Cover with pierced aluminium foil, and cook at 180°C (gas 4) for 12–15 minutes.
- Drain, season to taste, and serve immediately.

CARBOHYDRATE CONTENT PER SERVING: 3 GRAMS
(< 1 GRAM BY MICROWAVE METHOD)

Haddock with grilled Leerdammer

For 2
2 medium haddock fillets
100 ml full-cream milk
1 tbsp chopped fresh basil
1 tbsp chopped fresh coriander
2 slices pre-sliced Leerdammer cheese
freshly ground black pepper
2 large plum tomatoes on-the-vine, sliced

- Prepare the haddock according to the method (either baking or microwave) described above.

- Drain the haddock, sprinkle over the basil and coriander and top each fillet with a slice of Leerdammer cheese.
- Place under a hot grill for 30–40 seconds.
- Season to taste and serve with chopped tomato.

CARBOHYDRATE CONTENT PER SERVING: 6 GRAMS

Sardines with herbs

For 2
4 sardines (fresh or tinned)
1 tbsp chopped fresh basil (or 1 tsp dried basil)
1 tbsp chopped fresh coriander (or 1 tsp dried coriander)
juice of half a freshly squeezed lemon
freshly ground black pepper

- Grill the sardines under a hot grill (no closer than 8–10 cm from the grill) for 3–4 minutes, turning once.
- Remove from the grill, top with the herbs and sprinkle over the lemon juice.
- Return to the grill for a final 30 seconds, then season to taste and serve immediately.

CARBOHYDRATE CONTENT PER SERVING: 1 GRAM

Whiting with scrambled eggs and basil

For 2
4 small whiting fillets
2 large free-range eggs
1 tbsp chopped fresh basil
freshly ground black pepper
1 spring onion, finely diced

- Cook the whiting (pages 98–99) and prepare the scrambled eggs with basil (pages 85–86) as previously described.

- While the eggs are still slightly fluid, drain and flake the whiting, then stir the mixture into the scrambled eggs.
- Place the whiting and egg mixture in the microwave oven and cook on 'high' for a further 20 seconds.
- Serve immediately, season with freshly ground black pepper and garnish with spring onion.

CARBOHYDRATE CONTENT PER SERVING: 3 GRAMS

Smoked haddock with poached eggs

For 2
2 small smoked haddock fillets
pinch rock salt
2 large free-range eggs
pinch paprika
freshly ground black pepper

By microwave
- Place the smoked haddock fillets in a microwave-safe dish and cover.
- Cook on high for 2 minutes, then allow to stand for 1 minute.

Poached
- Place the smoked haddock fillets in a deep frying pan, add hot water to just cover the fillets and add a pinch of rock salt.
- Bring to the boil and reduce the heat to a gentle simmer for about 3–4 minutes.

At the same time
- Poach the eggs, either by microwave or conventional techniques (see pages 89–90).
- Carefully transfer the cooked haddock fillets with a

101

fish slice onto two warm plates, and place a poached egg on each haddock fillet.
- Sprinkle over a pinch of paprika and season with freshly ground black pepper.

CARBOHYDRATE CONTENT PER SERVING: NEGLIGIBLE

Mushrooms

Mushrooms can be cooked very quickly and make a delicious breakfast, either alone, or with a combination of herbs, tomatoes or bacon. An excellent source of vitamin B_2, mushrooms are also very nutritious. Button mushrooms are used in the following recipes as they have the lowest carbohydrate content, but different mushrooms have different flavours and you should use those you prefer. A delicious alternative is to mix together different varieties. The only type to absolutely avoid on a low-carb diet are shitake mushrooms which are very high in carbohydrates.

Mushrooms with bacon

This could be re-named 'the vitamin B breakfast': bacon is an excellent source of vitamin B_1 and mushrooms are an excellent source of vitamin B_2!

For 2
150 grams button mushrooms
50 grams butter
1 tbsp chopped fresh coriander
1 tbsp chopped fresh basil
4 rashers bacon
freshly ground black pepper

- Clean the mushrooms by wiping carefully, and remove the lower half-centimetre from the base of each stalk.
- Cut the button mushrooms in half lengthways.

- Heat the butter in a medium saucepan, and add the mushrooms.
- Cook for about 2 minutes, stirring frequently, then add the coriander and basil.
- Season to taste, and cook for a further 2 minutes.

At the same time
- Cook the bacon by microwave (or grill) for 3–4 minutes.
- Remove the mushroom and herb mixture with a perforated spoon, and serve with the bacon.

CARBOHYDRATE CONTENT PER SERVING: 1 GRAM

Tomatoes with mushrooms

Both tomatoes and herbs are rich sources of antioxidants and should be included in any healthy diet.

For 2
400 gram can plum tomatoes
1 tbsp chopped fresh oregano (or 1 tsp dried oregano)
1 tbsp chopped fresh coriander (or 1 tsp dried coriander)
50 grams butter
100 grams button mushrooms, wiped and halved lengthways
freshly ground black pepper

- Mix the herbs and tomatoes in a medium saucepan and heat thoroughly.
- Heat the butter in a shallow frying pan, sauté the mushrooms for approximately 2–3 minutes per side (depending on thickness), turning once.
- Serve the tomatoes with the mushrooms and season to taste with freshly ground black pepper.

CARBOHYDRATE CONTENT PER SERVING: 8 GRAMS

Avocado on toast

For 2

1 medium, ripe Hass avocado (peeled and stone
   removed), sliced
2 slices wholemeal bread, toasted
1 tsp Worcestershire sauce
freshly ground black pepper

- Spread the avocado slices over the toast.
- Drizzle over a few drops of Worcestershire sauce
  and season to taste.

CARBOHYDRATE CONTENT PER SERVING: 18 GRAMS

Bistro breakfast

Any of the following will provide a low-carbohydrate,
high-protein, nutritious breakfast, which is within the
guidelines for the diet.

Eggs cooked can be in the style you prefer and with
any low-carb accompaniment. Some examples would
include (but you are certainly not restricted to these
choices):

- Scrambled eggs on toast (one slice), possibly with
  herbs, spring onions or tomatoes
- Gammon steak
- Poached eggs, possibly with grilled tomatoes and
  mushrooms
- Eggs Benedict
- Bacon and mushrooms
- Omelettes (made with fresh free-range eggs), either
  plain, or with a selection of various low-
  carbohydrate fillings, such as:
    smoked salmon, finely chopped
    finely diced spring onion and Parma ham
    grated cheese (of choice): try Edam, Emmental
    or Bocconcini

fresh herbs, finely chopped: coriander parsley or chives
button mushrooms, sliced, then lightly fried in a little butter
cherry vine tomatoes, diced
shallots and basil

- Bacon and eggs (fried, poached or scrambled)
- Mushrooms on toast (single slice)
- Boiled eggs (up to 2), with a single slice of wholemeal toast
- Kippers with grilled tomatoes

Continental breakfast, consisting of a selection of cheeses, ham, sliced meats (such as salami, pastrami, pepperoni or chorizo), sliced chicken or turkey breast, smoked salmon or trout (with mayonnaise), avocado, tomatoes and a single piece of fruit (not banana). But definitely no cereals, pastries, pies, jams or croissants.

Take-away breakfast

Breakfast must be practical. Few of us have the luxury of a leisurely breakfast so we have to provide solutions to the problem of matching successful dieting with the practicalities of modern life. Actually, as you will see, it's really quite simple with just a little preparation. If it's simply not possible to have breakfast at home, or if you are one of the many people who simply cannot face food first thing in the morning, then we have to provide alternatives because the golden rule of successful weight loss is: *the diet has to fit your lifestyle, not the other way around.* If you try to adhere to a diet that is not suitable to your lifestyle it will inevitably fail. It is perfectly possible to adapt fast take-away food to this diet and to maintain healthy nutrition. Of course, it would be very difficult (but nevertheless possible) to obtain all the essential nutrients from a diet that was *entirely* based on take-away food, but there is certainly no reason why you can't eat out in the morning and still successfully diet and remain healthy. This diet caters for all situations.

You can have take-away breakfast in this diet but you have to prepare breakfast at home some mornings of the week, even if only at weekends, to ensure variety of diet and good nutrition. However, it needn't take much time to have a delicious breakfast which will sustain you until lunch, as you have already seen. And if you simply never have breakfast at home, you can obtain almost all the suggested home breakfast recipes in a deli or cafe – although obviously at greater expense.

The secret of having breakfast out and still losing weight easily, is to *select the appropriate choices from the menu.*

Even the take-away fast food in the 'traditional' sense can be included, providing you choose carefully. Naturally, because we are describing *how* you can enjoy breakfast in a typical 'fast food' outlet, it doesn't mean that we are advocating these outlets. The choice is yours. Sometimes you are left with little option; many of us have succumbed to our children's request for 'fast food' only to find ourselves perplexed as to what to choose from the menu and finally selecting a cup of coffee! Armed with the information in this book, you will now be able to select the 'healthiest' items from the take-away menu and still adhere to the diet.

The aim of this book is to provide as wide a choice as possible for all the different tastes and lifestyles that each of us enjoy as individuals. What we are trying to explain is that you can still eat nutritious and low-carb food in fast food outlets providing you choose carefully and omit the carbohydrates. Beef, chicken and salad is just as nutritious whether it is from McDonald's or the local gourmet restaurant! Examples of take-away fast foods which are low in carbohydrates include:

McDonald's breakfast

- Scrambled eggs (no muffin)
- Bacon and egg McMuffin (but discard the muffin)
- Sausage and egg McMuffin (discarding the muffin)
- Big breakfast (discarding the hash brown and muffin)

Definitely no hash browns, pancakes, muffins or jams. These are high in carbohydrate and must be avoided.

Drinks included:	tea
	decaf coffee
	all low-calorie soft drinks
Drinks excluded:	coffee
	all non low-calorie soft drinks
	all shakes
	orange juice

Burger King breakfast

All combinations of egg, cheese, sausage and bacon are included – provided you discard the bun or croissant. French toast is definitely out!

Drinks included:	tea
	decaf coffee
	all low-calorie soft drinks
Drinks excluded:	coffee
	all non low-calorie soft drinks
	all shakes
	orange juice

Take-away sandwiches

Breakfast on-the-run is not a good idea, either for lifestyle or health, as it is difficult for you to safely digest food whilst rushing around but, unfortunately, it is a fact of modern life for many of us and it has to be addressed if the diet is going to be successful. Circumstances often dictate our lifestyle and if we cannot adapt the diet to the individual lifestyle, it is

107

doomed to failure. The problem for most failed dieters is *not* willpower (which is a weak excuse from many other forms of diet for blaming the dieter for failure instead of an impossible low-calorie diet); but *lack of choice*. As we all know, almost all fast foods instantly available are essentially high-carb foods: sandwiches, ciabatta, panini, baguettes, tortillas, to name but a few of the myriad high-carb snacks available. And the reason is simply that bread products are the only easy way to handle and transport food. In many ways, the Earl of Sandwich has much to answer for regarding the effect his 'discovery' has had on the health of subsequent generations!

It is, quite simply, very difficult to hold and consume a bacon sandwich without the bread! For a moment, pause to consider how you can overcome this problem in your own situation because essentially that is the cause of the difficulty. The *contents* of most sandwiches are usually of a very high standard nutritionally, it is the *bread* which causes the problem with a low-carb diet.

The solution is very simple. As we have already explained, most fillings of sandwiches are very healthy and nutritious (for example, egg mayonnaise, ham and cheese, bacon/lettuce/tomato, to name a very few of the almost infinite array of possibilities), so you need to order a sandwich with a large filling to satisfy your appetite. You can carry the sandwich to wherever you intend to enjoy your breakfast, then discard the upper layer of bread (which contributes little to the meal either gastronomically or nutritionally) and enjoy the 'open' sandwich. If it is a 'hot' or 'messy' meal (for example, egg mayonnaise), you should request a set of disposable cutlery from the take-away outlet or, to be absolutely certain, just carry a set yourself in case of emergencies. The basis of successful low-carb dieting is to think and act in a totally different way. At present, the structure of our eating habits is totally geared to the carbohydrate culture because carbohydrate foods are easy to produce cheaply! With just a little forethought and preparation, not just in the food you buy but also in the way you think, it is very easy to beat the carbohydrate traps that modern life sets and diet successfully in virtually every situation. Typical 'breakfast sandwiches' which would easily conform with your diet include all of the usual breakfast options, such as:

- bacon
- egg mayonnaise
- scrambled egg
- bacon, lettuce and tomato
- sausage
- sausage and egg
- egg and tomato

Remember you don't need to keep to the typical breakfast: providing you keep to a low-carb option, you can enjoy any alternative style of food. The following are potential delicious variations on the usual breakfast fare which are generally available from take-away outlets and delicatessens:

- chicken and bacon
- feta cheese with olives and Lebanese cucumber
- mushrooms with red peppers and a drizzle of extra-virgin olive oil
- egg and tomato with mayonnaise
- Emmental cheese with Parma ham
- smoked salmon with mayonnaise
- mozzarella cheese with sliced plum tomato and balsamic vinegar
- chicken with mayonnaise
- avocado and tomato
- Gruyere with mixed salad
- pastrami with wholegrain mustard

We will provide a simple answer to explain how to carry an open sandwich on page 153.

Chapter 6

Lunch

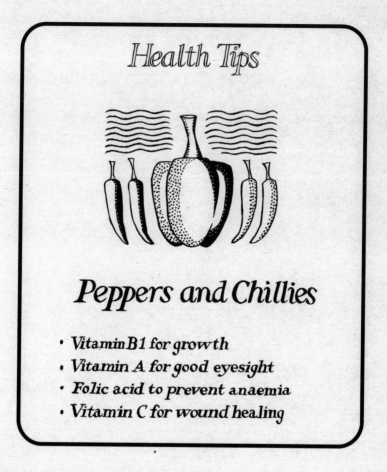

Health Tips

Peppers and Chillies

- *Vitamin B1 for growth*
- *Vitamin A for good eyesight*
- *Folic acid to prevent anaemia*
- *Vitamin C for wound healing*

Salad lunchboxes

Chicken breast with chilli sauce	143–44
Egg mayonnaise with fresh basil and chives	144–45
Roast ham with Leerdammer cheese and mustard	145
Avocado with Bocconcini cheese	146
Tuna mayonnaise with basil and coriander	146–47
Roast beef and pickle	147
Salmon with crème fraîche	147–48
Greek salad	148–49
Chicken with curry and herb sauce	149–50
Tiger prawns with chilli and coriander vinaigrette	150–51
Tiger prawns with lemon and coriander vinaigrette	151
Port Salut, courgettes and chives salad	151–52

Sandwiches

Chicken with mayonnaise and avocado open sandwich	155
Ham, eggs and chives open sandwich	155–56
Prawn mayonnaise open sandwich	156
Tuna mayonnaise open sandwich	156–57
Bacon lettuce and tomato open sandwich	157–58
Crab salad open sandwich	158
Salsa steak open sandwich	158–59
Salami salad open sandwich	159

Lunch at home

Hot-and-spicy chicken drumsticks with baby spinach leaves	160–61
Haddock with herbs	162–63
Gammon steaks with balsamic vinegar	163
Smoked trout with avocado	163–64
Spicy prawns with rocket	164–65
Tandoori lamb with cucumber raita	165

Tuna with spinach and basil 165–66
Savoury crêpes 166–68
Hoisin duck crêpes 168
Prawn mayonnaise crêpes 169
Spinach and Emmental crêpes 169–70
Cod with orange sauce 170–71
Steak with asparagus purée 171–72
Chargrilled Madras sardines with crème
 fraîche 172

Lunch is easy to plan around a low-carb diet, whatever your lifestyle, because the array of choices available from supermarkets and delicatessens of low-carb foods (which also happen to be highly nutritious foods) is simply immense. But these are not the foods you immediately associate with the term 'fast food', which has really been hijacked by the carbohydrate industry. When you mention fast food, you immediately think of sandwiches, burgers, fast-food outlets such as McDonald's, Burger King and Kentucky Fried Chicken, Chinese take-away, Indian take-away, kebabs . . . Most of these 'fast foods' are just another term for 'high-carb' foods but even many of these can be easily adapted to a low-carb lifestyle. For example, if you discard the bun of a McDonald's Quarterpounder, you have instantaneously converted a high-carb (and therefore fattening) meal into a low-carb (and therefore slimming) meal. The beef is of high quality and the salad packed with additional nutrients.

Exactly the same principle applies to many so-called 'fast' foods. When you remove the carbohydrate part of the meal, the remainder is actually full of nutrients and perfectly suitable for a diet. In Kentucky Fried Chicken, for example, remove the batter coating and you are left with pure chicken packed with all the essential amino acids you need to build body protein. Of course we are not suggesting you live on 'fast foods' or even that you *ever* indulge in the typical 'fast' food, but it merely demonstrates how easily some of them can be converted from highly fattening food to nutritious food suitable for a low-carb diet. Naturally, some fast foods are incapable of being healthy, mainly those where most of the food is actually carbohydrate (such as pies, sausage rolls, pasties, pasta, white rice and chips).

The phrase *the secret of successful dieting is planning* is repeatedly quoted throughout this book because the only way to prevent the diet failing is by always having low-carb foods available. This is especially important in relation to lunch when we are bombarded with a vast array of take-away foods, most of which are totally unsuitable to any form of diet, especially a low-carb diet, as they consist mainly of carbohydrates (which are a cheap alternative to *real* nutritious food). There are many delicious foods available that are ideal for a take-away lunch, but unless you know which to choose, you will inevitably be caught in the high-carb lunch trap because there is seemingly nothing else available. Nothing could be further from the truth! But you have to learn to think in a different way. The outlets that you usually associated with take-away food have some foods which can be adapted to a low-carb diet, but not many. We have already described how a McDonald's Quarterpounder and Kentucky Fried Chicken can be easily adapted and we will provide many more examples of similar foods.

The best source of excellent take-away fast foods are certainly not the 'normal' take-away fast-food outlets. In fact, the most appropriate fast foods are available in immense variety from supermarkets (including Marks and Spencer) and delicatessens. If you have a microwave at work you can enjoy foods as diverse as Cottage pie (19 grams of carbohydrate), Prawn salad with seafood sauce (20 grams of carbohydrate) or Chicken curry (14 grams of carbohydrate), all of which can be easily incorporated into a low-carb fast food diet – and all of which are also highly nutritious.

For practical purposes we have subdivided the lunch chapter into five separate categories, corresponding to the most common practices at lunch:

- Take-away lunch – cold
- Take-away lunch – hot
- Packed lunch
- Lunch at home
- Bistro lunch

Each of the categories has been divided into 'Foods to be included' and 'Foods to be avoided', however, in many instances, the same outlets are represented in both categories. In effect, this is the essence of the book, because it will explain which foods are to be included *from whatever food outlet* and which are to be excluded. It is not as simple as pontificating that 'you must eat here' and 'you must not eat there'. In fact, with very few exceptions, you can enjoy most foods, providing the refined carbohydrates are removed. And as the combination of carbohydrates with trans fats is probably the unhealthiest possible combination, when you remove refined carbohydrates from the meal the remaining constituents are usually highly nutritious!

Take-away lunch – cold

Probably the most frequent lunch for those away from home at lunch-time is the 'cold' take-away. You can obtain food which is low-carb (with a little adaptation) from the typical take-away outlet but by far the best (and widest selection) of low-carb food is obtained from supermarkets and delicatessens.

The single most important 'emergency' low-carb food at lunchtime is chicken. Why 'emergency'? Because everyone on a low-carb diet will have a low-carb 'emergency' at lunchtime at one time or another, surrounded by the plethora of high-carb foods which make up the basis of the current take-away lunch market and will be unsure of how to select something low-carb and 'safe'. Look for the nearest supermarket (there is almost always one nearby) and search out the cooked meats section. Cooked chicken is sold in many different ways: as slices of chicken breast (which is not particularly appropriate or satisfying at lunch) or as breast, thighs, wings or drumsticks, either plain or in a variety of sauces, most of which are very low in carbohydrates and therefore ideal for a low-carb diet. Some of the many sauces available include barbecue, tikka and Chinese. The average carbohydrate content of chicken marinated in these sauces is about 2 grams per hundred grams, which in practical terms equates to 1–2 grams of carbohydrate per chicken drumstick (depending on the size of the drumstick), effectively almost negligible. These can be enjoyed without accompaniment, are ready-prepared and relatively inexpensive, can be consumed immediately, taste delicious and, most importantly, *satisfy the most voracious appetite almost immediately.*

Supermarkets, take-away outlets and delicatessens are probably the sources of most working lunches today. They are also the likeliest place you will go when in a hurry at lunchtime so it is important to be aware of how to maintain your low-carb diet on the choices available. There are a wide variety of different meals available from supermarkets and it is important to include Marks and Spencer in this category as it doesn't really fit any other specific category.

In general, particularly with supermarkets and Marks and Spencer, the best advice is *avoid the take-away section and head straight for the deli foods.* Take-away foods in these outlets essentially mean high-carb foods, with various sandwiches, tortilla wraps, ciabatta, paninis, bagels and French breads. Even seemingly healthy low-carb meals such as tuna-layered salad have hidden dangers; as you know, tuna and salad are very low-carb foods but they can be mixed with pasta which ruins the diet. You have to be constantly vigilant for hidden carbohydrates. The most common culprit is the 'hidden' pasta, often buried beneath salad in an otherwise delicious meal. Another typical example is a prawn salad, which has prawns, seafood sauce and salad (all low-carb) on a base of pasta shells (very high-carb!). The secret is either to leave the pasta, or buy something else.

So the only choices available in the take-away sections of these outlets are:

(a) Purchase sandwiches or wraps with low-carb fillings (meat, fish, chicken, mayonnaise, salad, vegetables, eggs or cheese) and consume only the filling. Very impractical as most of the meal is actually the bread (in whatever form) and this will not leave you satisfied and is certainly not economical. In this diet it is the *filling* which is low-carb and you really should have sandwiches with a considerable filling so that you can discard the upper slice of bread and enjoy an open sandwich. Sandwiches are best purchased from a take-away sandwich outlet or delicatessen where you can specify the kind and amount of filling. You can then easily afford to discard the upper layer of bread and still have a satisfying open sandwich for lunch.

(b) Purchase the pasta salads (such as prawn salad or tuna salad) and consume the seafood and salad but leave the pasta.

Neither of these choices is particularly satisfactory but fortunately they are unnecessary as the solution to the problem lies in the deli section. Deli foods are absolutely perfect for a low-carb diet as they are almost all low-carb. Added to the fact that they are usually packed with healthy nutrients (primarily because they are low in carbohydrates) and you have the perfect healthy 'fast food' lunch. Also, they are pre-packed in suitable sealed containers so they can be easily transported to wherever you intend to enjoy your lunch. Always carry some disposable cutlery and a paper napkin and your only limiting factor in maintaining your low-carb take-away lunch will be the proximity of the nearest supermarket or delicatessen!

A word of caution. The nutritional content of similar products varies from one supermarket to another so, to repeat once again, you must read the nutritional label to check the carbohydrate content. A barbecue sauce may be very low-carb in one outlet and contain more sugar in another.

Supermarkets have a common habit of changing the nature of the products available, so while this list is accurate at the present time it could change overnight. That is not a problem for the educated low-carb dieter. Supermarkets usually replace one product with another similar product (for example one chicken sauce with another) so providing you acquire the habit of *always reading the nutritional product label* you can be certain to enjoy safe low-carb ready-cooked foods without the danger of ruining your low-carb diet.

Some examples of delicious foods which would be eminently suitable for a low-carb diet are as follows. The gram-weights have been rounded to approximate figures for simplicity.

Supermarket deli take-away foods included in the diet virtually without restriction

Food	Weight (g)	Carbs (g)		Protein (g)	
		per pack	per 100g	per pack	per 100g
Caesar salad	290	2	1	7	5
Tomato and mozzarella cheese salad	220	7	3	22	10
Egg mayonnaise	170	<1	<1	17	10

Food	Weight (g)	Carbs (g) per pack	Carbs (g) per 100g	Protein (g) per pack	Protein (g) per 100g
Prawn mayonnaise	170	< 1	< 1	18	11
Smoked salmon and soft cheese	170	8	5	18	11
Chicken and sweetcorn	170	7	4	21	12
Chicken liver pâté	170	3	2	21	12
Tuna pâté	170	< 1	< 1	21	12
Brussels pâté	170	5	3	22	13
Duck and orange pâté	170	7	4	17	10
Spicy salmon	170	10	6	3	2
Sour cream and chives	170	6	4	5	3
Kalamata olives	180	4	2	4	2
Meze selection	580				

In meze, some are included (olives, tzatziki, taramasalata) whilst others are excluded (Falafel, stuffed vine leaves or houmous).

Food	Weight (g)	Carbs (g) per pack	Carbs (g) per 100g	Protein (g) per pack	Protein (g) per 100g
Olives			4		1
Tsatziki			6		6
Taramasalata			6		5
Falafel			19		8
Stuffed vine leaves			13		3
Houmus			8		8
Scotch eggs	120	18	15	14	12
'Mini' Scotch egg (each)	18	3	15	14	12
Dressed lobster	180	2	1	25	14

Food	Weight (g)	Carbs (g)		Protein (g)	
		per pack	per 100g	per pack	per 100g
Poached salmon fillets	200	< 1	< 1	44	22
Dressed crab	125	11	9	21	17
Prawn cocktail	200	4	2	18	9
Coleslaw	400	16	4	4	1
Cooked tiger prawns	140	< 1	< 1	25	18
Crab pâté	115	7	6	14	12
Smoked mackerel pâté	115	1	1	18	16
Tuna and sweetcorn mayonnaise	340	7	2	45	14
Egg and sweet-cured bacon with mayo	170	5	3	24	14
King prawns with salsa	200	2	1	24	12
Egg and onion mayo	170	5	3	17	10
Chicken, tomato, sweetcured bacon with mayonnaise	170	5	3	11	19
Salmon terrine with prawn and lobster	170	7	4	31	18
Chilli and coriander prawns	140	< 1	< 1	31	18

Probably the most convenient very low-carb food which is readily available pre-packaged (and therefore easily transported) from supermarkets is cooked chicken, which is very low-carb, whether as breast, drumsticks, thighs or wings. It can be safely included in the diet either plain or with a tasty sauce but you must read the nutrition label to check the carbohydrate content as some sauces are high in carbohydrates.

The perfect cold take-away has virtually no (or an insignificant amount) of carbohydrate, *and this does exist!* You can enjoy virtually unlimited quantities of all meats and cheeses in your diet which are easily obtainable from the deli section in supermarkets. This includes roast beef, hams, salamis, cooked turkey and all varieties of pure (i.e. not processed) cheese.

Cooked chicken included without restriction on a low-carb diet

Food	Carbs (g) per 100g	Protein (g) per 100g
Chicken (breast, drumsticks, thighs, wings):		
Plain	< 1	24
Tikka sauce	< 1	24
Barbecue	2	24
Chicken breast:		
Tomato and basil sauce	2	23
Sweet chilli and lime sauce	3	26
Tex Mex	< 1	23
Chicken kebabs		
Chinese sauce	5	27
Tikka	< 1	24
Tex Mex	< 1	26

Cooked chicken with some restrictions (i.e. < 200 g per serving)

Food	Carb (g) per 100g	Protein (g) per 100g
Coronation chicken	10	12
Chinese chicken	7	20

Cooked chicken excluded from the diet

Hot and spicy chicken	16	20

Supermarket deli take-away foods which can be included in a low-carb diet, omitting the carbohydrates

The following foods are only high-carb because the meal is placed on a bed of pasta. Leave out the pasta and the meal becomes very nutritious and very low in carbohydrates; however the most nutritious foods are those described above where the entire meal can be consumed.

Food	Weight (g)	Carbs (g) per 100g	Protein (g) per 100g
Tuna layered salad (tuna, carrot, cucumber sweet corn pasta)	450	8	7
Prawn layered salad	450	10	4
Honey and mustard chicken with pasta	190	17	8

Similarly, quiche can be converted from a high-carb meal to a very low-carb (and highly nutritious) meal by simply consuming the filling and leaving the pastry casing:

Food	Weight (g)	Carbs (g) per 100g	Protein (g) per 100g
Quiche:			
Lorraine	400	15	11
Cheese and			
Tomato	400	15	8
Broccoli and			
Tomato	400	14	6

Take-away sandwich outlets

Providing you only have one slice of bread (discarding the upper layer), the low-carb sandwich filling will incur a maximum of 20 grams of carbohydrate for lunch (15–17 grams from the single slice of bread alone). It is the *filling* which is healthy, not the bread, so stock up on a large filling for the sandwich and you will not be hungry later. Obviously it is very difficult to carry an open sandwich (although we will explain how this *can* easily be achieved with open sandwiches from home on page 153) so the easiest solution is to have a normal take-away sandwich with a (preferably) large and delicious filling, then discard the upper layer of bread and consume the sandwich with disposable plastic cutlery (which is available from most take-away outlets).

There is a wide variety of take-away outlets which provide sandwiches and sandwich-style products, from small sandwich bars to supermarkets. In supermarkets your choice of sandwich is obviously limited to those available, so you have to choose a low-carb filling from the selection but you have no opportunity to increase the *amount* of the filling. In take-away sandwich outlets and delicatessens, however, you can usually select your own filling or combination of fillings so it is relatively simple to enjoy extra low-carb filling which replaces the bread (thereby preventing hunger) and achieves the perfect solution of promoting healthy weight loss with relatively little effort on the part of the dieter (the dieter's dream!).

In summary, take-away sandwiches for lunch are best purchased from take-away sandwich outlets and delicatessens where you can control the amount of the filling, rather than from supermarkets where you have no control over the amount of pre-packaged sandwich filling.

Typical fillings would include (but are certainly not restricted to):

Prawn mayonnaise
Ham, cheese (of multiple varieties) and pickle
Chicken salad
Chicken, salsa and avocado
Steak salad
Egg and cress
Chicken and bacon
Smoked ham and mustard
Salmon and cucumber
Roasted peppers and sun-dried tomatoes
Ploughman's, with Cheddar cheese, pickle and onions
Roast beef and horseradish sauce
Cheese and celery with mayonnaise
Tuna mayonnaise
Egg and prawns
Avocado, mozzarella and sun-dried tomatoes
Poached salmon (with or without mayonnaise)
Chicken tikka
Roast pork with apple sauce
Smoked turkey breast with cranberry sauce
Emmental cheese with honey ham
Chargrilled peppers with chicken breast
Mozzarella, plum tomato and balsamic vinegar
Egg mayonnaise
Bacon, lettuce and tomato

Avocado with tomato and mayonnaise
Coronation chicken with green salad

And don't forget that many take-away sandwich outlets
also provide salad boxes with fillings of choice. This is
really the perfect solution to the problem of the low-
carb take-away lunch as the absence of bread (or pasta
or rice) means that this is virtually no-carb rather than
low-carb. The basis of the 'box' is a salad of choice –
with either vinaigrette or mayonnaise, of course – and,
providing you keep to high protein foods, the
possibilities are almost infinite. Obviously all the above
sandwich fillings are suitable for the salad box, which is
provided with disposable cutlery and napkins and is a
perfect low-carb take-away. With all these delicious
fillings in virtually unlimited quantities, this low-carb
diet is certainly not an ordeal!

The choices in either open sandwiches or preferably
salad boxes are really only limited by your personal
preferences. There is a considerable overlap between
meals; many of the same choices are equally suitable
for breakfast, lunch or light supper. The route to
success in dieting is to *think about food in a completely
different way, and plan your meals accordingly.*

Delicatessen
Deli foods are perfect for a low-carb diet because
almost all their foods are naturally low in
carbohydrates: salami, cooked hams/beef/chicken,
cheeses (usually of immense variety) and prepared
mixtures of delicious foods. In addition to the
possibility of sandwiches with multiple fillings (which
can then be converted to an open sandwich by
discarding the upper layer of bread when you have
arrived at your destination), there are also many
choices of delicious prepared foods which can be
purchased in medium containers and consumed using

disposable cutlery supplied by the deli. Salad boxes, similar to those described from take-away sandwich outlets, are usually available with similar fillings of high protein, very low-carb foods.

Every delicatessen is unique in the foods they prepare; however, the following will provide a guide to some of the many foods which can be included in a low-carb diet, and those which must be avoided.

Deli foods which can be included in a low-carb diet

Coronation chicken – in moderation
Egg mayonnaise
Chicken tikka
Olives
Herrings – in sherry
              in dill sauce
              sweet cured
              'roll mops'
Tuna mayonnaise
Farmer salad (coleslaw)
German meat salad
Mozzarella, sundried tomatoes, basil and mayonnaise
Taramasalata
Prawn mayonnaise
Emmental cheese, bacon and mayonnaise
Aubergine pâté
Chicken and sundried tomatoes
Mixed cheese, leek and onion salad
Red pepper and sundried tomato salad
Chicken, bacon and mayonnaise
Italian chicken
Sundried tomatoes
Artichokes in olive oil
Chicken liver pâté

These are all low-carb and, therefore, eminently

suitable for the diet. There are so many delicatessens that you never seem to be far from one – a completely new dimension to the concept of 'convenience food'.

Of course there are also some deli foods which, although healthy, cannot be included in a low-carb diet, especially those with pulses and grain products:

Deli foods which cannot be included in a low-carb diet
Spinach, feta cheese and lentil pâté
Any filling with sweetcorn
Sundried tomatoes and lentil pâté
Spicy bean pâté
Tabboulah salad
Hummus

Subway
Subway sandwich outlets are ubiquitous and provide an excellent example of how to customise your lunch to a low-carb, healthy diet. The bread is ideal for allowing you to transport the healthy contents, but for little else. Fill the sandwich with healthy fillings (listed below), then discard the upper layer of bread and enjoy an open sandwich. It is probably best to carry disposable cutlery as a large open sandwich can be a little difficult to eat without it. The bread roll is quite large and even half a roll may contain as many as 20 grams of carbohydrate, so if you can enjoy your meal without bread simply consume the filling alone, which should reduce the carbohydrates to 6–8 grams; with the lower half of the roll, the total carbohydrate content would be 26–28 grams, on average.

Sandwiches have a base of salad such as lettuce, tomatoes, onions, peppers, olives, pickles, cheese, oil, vinegar and seasoning.

Typical fillings of a Subway sandwich include seafood, tuna, ham, roast beef, cheese and turkey, all of which are excellent sources of essential amino acids. Avoid the bread, and you can continue to enjoy your low-carb healthy diet at Subway.

Cold take-away foods to be avoided on a low-carb diet

General guidelines for foods which must be avoided are those which have obvious carbohydrates, such as rice, pasta and bread.

Supermarkets

Sushi, pasta salads and sandwiches are out, but, of course, you can discard the upper layer of bread in the sandwich, converting it to an open sandwich.

Foods which are absolutely excluded from the diet are those comprising mainly carbohydrates where the nutritious component cannot be separated from the carbohydrates.

Meals which are relatively high in carbohydrates, to be avoided, include:

Food	Weight (g)	Carbs (g) per 100g	Protein (g) per 100g
Couscous and chargrilled vegetables	200	23	4
Hummus	280	8	7
Fish sushi	210	25	6
Vegetable sushi	210	25	4
Moroccan spiced carrot salad	200	14	4

- **Pizza**

  The base of a pizza is about 73% pure carbohydrate and you can't get much more high-carb than that. A quarter slice of an average pizza contains approximately 30 grams of carbohydrate. It is actually possible to include pizza in a low-carb diet, but only if you eat the topping (which is low-carb and actually nutritious) and discard all of the base. As very few of us would have the willpower to discard all of the base, pizza is definitely best avoided on a low-carb diet.

- **Pasta and noodles**
Like pizza base, pasta and noodles are virtually pure carbohydrate so **all** pastas are excluded from the diet. Although the pasta in spaghetti and lasagna is very obviously present, many foods have 'hidden' pastas: pre-packaged salads are often served with a base of pasta which increases the carbohydrate content of the meal immensely. Always read the carbohydrate content of any pre-packaged foods, and look for the hidden pasta. You can still enjoy the meal by simply not consuming the pasta! And definitely no 'pot noodle-style' foods.

- **Almost all flour-based products: breads/rolls/tortillas/ciabatta/panini/baguettes/naan/bagels . . .**
These are all very high in carbohydrates, especially the more unleavened varieties like tortillas, ciabatta, bagels and naan bread. A single bagel or tortilla can contain up to 30 grams of carbohydrate, depending on size. As previously explained, you *can* include a sandwich in the diet, providing you discard the top slice of bread to create an open sandwich, thereby reducing your carbohydrate intake from 30–34 grams to 15–17 grams. Most fillings are either low-carb (like salad) or no-carb (like meat, chicken, cheese, eggs, fish and shellfish), so you can enjoy

more filling (which is the tastiest part of the sandwich) and less bread.

- **Pies/sausage rolls/pasties**
  A large proportion of the content is carbohydrate and fats, the worst possible combination. The carbohydrates stimulate insulin to convert most of the calories to body fat, exactly the situation you are trying to avoid.

- **Cakes/biscuits/croissants/pastries**
  Once again, the deadly combination of carbohydrates and fats, guaranteed to be deposited immediately on your waist and hips. Definitely to be avoided.

- **All chocolates and confectionary**
  Very high in sugar content and guaranteed to return the sugar addiction and ruin your diet.

- **All potato crisps**
  The worst possible combination of carbohydrates and fats which will be immediately deposited on your waist (for men) and hips and thighs (for women).

Take-away lunch – hot
Hot take-away foods which can be safely included in a low-carb diet

- **Shish kebabs**
  Shish kebabs are the perfect low-carb, high nutrition meal – providing you discard the bread. Usually there is a substantial filling of lean meat and salad providing many essential amino acids, vitamins and minerals – and virtually no carbohydrates.

McDonald's

Although you probably never expected to find McDonald's in a diet book, and especially not a diet book with the aim of promoting health and nutrition, many of the McDonald's high-carb meals can actually be easily adapted to low-carb by removing the offending carbohydrates. As we have already seen, a Quarterpounder is full of essential amino acids and the tomato and salad provides other essential vitamins and minerals. But to include this in your diet you have remove the carbohydrate part of the meal – the bun. Strange though it may seem, the bun is actually the unhealthiest part of the meal as it consists mainly of carbohydrates (about 27 grams of carbohydrates), with virtually no carbohydrates in the burger and salad. So providing you remove the bun, you have instantly created a nutritious low-carb meal. Remember, the fat in a meal will not be deposited as body fat unless you also consume carbohydrates because carbohydrates control the body's deposition of fat.

Having explained how easy it is to convert some – but not all – McDonald's meals into a low-carb alternative, you can now appreciate how this can be adapted to other meals. It is our aim to provide you with the *principles* of the diet, not every possible variation; once you understand the *concepts* you can easily decide for yourself foods which are healthy and low-carb, and those which definitely are not! Remove the buns from these meals, and you effectively convert them to low-carb:

Quarterpounder
Quarterpounder with cheese
Big Mac
McChicken
Filet-o-Fish
Cheeseburger

Double cheeseburger
Hamburger

Low-carb drinks which you can enjoy with your low-carb meal include tea, decaf coffee and all diet drinks.

Although these items from McDonald's are definitely very low-carb, are they healthy? The answer, surprising though it may seem, is 'yes'! To explain this in more detail, we will examine the ingredients (obtained from McDonald's official website) in each of the above meals, and their nutritional significance. But please don't misunderstand the intention of this information. We certainly do not advocate a diet based on typical fast foods, as they contain other undesirable elements (such as 'trans' fats and preservatives) but merely to demonstrate that you can obtain much needed essential nutrition even from the 'typical' fast foods, and you can still lose weight on a low-carb diet if you omit certain of the menu items and all of the buns!

But always remember that fresh food, without preservatives, is much healthier, so if you have to visit a fast food outlet, choose carefully and try to limit your visits. Armed with the information in this book, you can easily increase the amount of 'fresh' fast foods in your diet at the expense of the 'typical' fast foods, even if you don't have either the time or inclination to cook!

- **Quarterpounder with cheese**
  with bun: total carbs 38 grams
  without bun: total carbs 7 grams

  Nutritional value: 100% beef patty (provides all essential amino acids), cheese (essential amino acids and vitamin D), tomato ketchup (vitamin A and the antioxidant lycopene), mustard (antioxidants from the spices and sulphur from mustard), pickle (vitamin A from cucumber) and onions (an excellent source of natural antioxidants).

You can see that if you remove the bun, you reduce the carbohydrate content to only 7 grams, and the remaining ingredients are nutritious.

- **Big Mac**
  with bun: total carbs 47 grams
  without bun: total carbs 11 grams

  Contents and nutritional value are similar (but not identical) to a quarterpounder.

- **Filet-o-Fish**
  with bun: total carbs 45 grams
  without bun: total carbs 16 grams

  Nutritional value: essential amino acids from the fish, antioxidants from the mustard and onions in the tartare sauce, and vitamin D and calcium from the cheese.

- **McChicken**
  with bun: total carbs 41 grams
  without bun: total carbs 12 grams

  Nutritional value: essential amino acids from chicken, vitamins D and B_{12} from the eggs in the mayonnaise and vitamin A from lettuce.

Meals and drinks to be avoided (on a low-carb diet) at McDonald's are basically everything else on the menu, many of which are described on pages 130–140.

Burger King
Exactly the same principles apply to Burger King as to McDonald's. The beef contains virtually no carbohydrates,

which are almost all restricted to the bun. For example, a Double Whopper contains 52 grams of carbohydrates, of which 45 grams are from the bun alone! So if you discard the bun, the meal contains only 7 grams of carbohydrates. And as the burger patties are made from 100% pure beef, it can hardly be considered unhealthy. Once again, it is not our intention to list *all* the menu items, but rather to provide you with guidelines of those you may include in your diet, and those to avoid.

Items from the Burger King menu which can be easily included in your low-carb diet are as follows. Remember you *must* discard the bun for the item to become low-carb; with the bun, it is very *high-carb*!

Whopper
Double Whopper
Double Whopper with cheese
Hamburger
Cheeseburger
Bacon cheeseburger
Bacon double cheeseburger
Chicken Whopper

Some examples of the carbohydrate content (with and without the bun) of typical Burger King menu items are as follows. This information was obtained from the official Burger King website.

- **Whopper with cheese**
  with bun: total carbs 50 grams
  without bun: total carbs 5 grams

  Nutritional value: the contents of the Whopper are listed as 100% beef patty (providing essential amino acids), tomatoes (antioxidant lycopene), cheese (vitamin D and calcium), lettuce (vitamin A), pickles (vitamin A), mayonnaise (vitamins D and B_{12}) and ketchup (antioxidant lycopene).

- **Bacon double cheeseburger**
  with bun: total carbs 33 grams
  without bun: total carbs 5 grams

  Nutritional value: beef patty (essential amino acids), cheese (vitamin D and calcium), pickles (vitamin A), ketchup (antioxidant lycopene), bacon (essential amino acids and vitamin B_1) and mustard (excellent source of the mineral sulphur).

- **Chicken Whopper**
  with bun: total carbs 32 grams
  without bun: total carbs: 4 grams

  Nutritional value: boiled chicken fillet (essential amino acids), tomatoes (vitamin A and lycopene), lettuce (folic acid) and mayonnaise (vitamins D and B_{12}).

Kentucky Fried Chicken

The situation with Kentucky Fried Chicken is slightly different, as many of the meals do not use buns but rather batter on the chicken. The principles of the low-carb diet remains the same: remove the offending carbohydrates (in this case batter) and the underlying chicken is delicious and nutritious, providing all the essential amino acids for our daily protein requirements. So you can enjoy any of the 'pure' chicken meals (like 'Original recipe', or 'Hot and Spicy') either as breast, wings or drumsticks, *providing you remove and discard all the batter*. Almost all the carbohydrate content is contained within the batter; remove the batter and you have a low-carb meal. But have none of the KFC sandwiches which are relatively high in carbohydrates.

Hot take-away foods which must be avoided on a low-carb diet

Many of the cold take-away foods to be avoided can also be served hot, so you will notice an overlap, however it is important to ensure there is no doubt regarding which foods are to be totally excluded from your diet.

- Pizza
- Pasta and noodles
- Almost all flour-based products: breads/rolls/tortillas/ciabatta/panini/baguettes/naan/bagels, which can also be served heated or toasted
- Pies/sausage rolls/pasties

Other foods which must be avoided include:

- **Chips**
  Potato contains a relatively high proportion of carbohydrates, and the combination of carbohydrates and fat is the perfect combination to make you fat, so chips are definitely excluded.

- **Soups**
  Home-made soup is perfectly acceptable on a low-carb diet because you know what is in it! Unfortunately that is not the case with take-away soup which often may be high in 'hidden' carbohydrates, so you have to exclude this from your diet. If you intend to include convenience foods in your diet it is essential to be sure that they don't contain too much carbohydrate which will ruin the diet. Carbohydrates (especially sugar) are a very common ingredient in many convenience foods as they are very cheap and quite addictive, which is a perfect combination for the take-away industry!

- **Most fried foods**
  Most take-away fried foods are high in carbohydrate content and trans fats, so they must be excluded.

- **Baked potato**
  Potato has a high carbohydrate content and must be excluded during the weight loss phase, although baked potatoes are healthy (with a healthy concentration of vitamin C) and can be re-introduced to your diet after the weight loss phase. Most of the fillings in baked potatoes from take-away outlets are actually low in carbohydrate content.

Chinese take-away

Chinese food prepared at home can be very healthy and nutritious. We will provide recipes for Chinese food which can be made quickly at home but are more suitable for dinner, particularly in terms of the time required for preparation. Chinese take-away can also be low in carbohydrates, but unfortunately many meals have hidden carbohydrates and sugars, so you have to avoid them as you don't know their content. Obviously rice and noodles are absolutely excluded from the diet.

Indian take-away

Indian foods are very healthy, nutritious and suitable for a low-carb diet, however take-away ready-cooked foods can have hidden sugars added, so they must be avoided. But you can buy delicious prepared Indian meals from supermarkets (including Marks and Spencer) which are low in carbohydrates; the carbohydrate content of different foods is clearly listed on the label. Each supermarket produces its own range of meals and they all differ in carbohydrate content, so you must acquire the habit of reading the label to be sure that the meal has a low carbohydrate content.

A list of supermarket foods which are suitable is

provided on pages 120–23. Those supermarket foods which must be avoided (as they are relatively high in carbohydrates) are described on pages 130–32. The golden rule is *always* read the carbohydrate content in the nutritional information on each package. This will tell you the carbohydrate content of the entire meal, and give you an instant answer as to whether you can include the meal in your diet or leave it on the shelf! If in doubt, leave it on the shelf.

McDonald's
As we have explained, some McDonald's meals can be included in a low-carb diet easily – and provide excellent nutrition – but others must be totally excluded for their high carbohydrate content.

- **Meals which must be excluded are:**
  Buns
  French fries
  Chicken McNuggets
  Shakes
  Desserts
  Non-diet soft drinks
  Orange juice

Burger King
Items to be excluded are very similar to those in the McDonald's Menu:

- **Meals which must be excluded are:**
  Buns
  French fries
  Onion rings
  Chicken tenders
  Shakes
  Desserts
  Non-diet soft drinks

Kentucky Fried Chicken

- **Items to be definitely excluded are:**
  Sandwiches
  Buns
  Batter on chicken
  French fries
  Vegetables/coleslaw
  Desserts
  Non-diet soft drinks

Packed lunch

Many of these meals can be equally applied to either light lunch at home, or late suppers, so there is substantial overlap between the chapters. The only absolutely essential prerequisite is that you keep to low-carb food which is healthy!

Few packed lunches can be successfully prepared the previous evening because the taste 16 hours later is definitely not good. Essentially our choices fall into the following general categories:

- Salad lunchbox – with an infinite array of possibilities
- Sandwiches – especially open sandwiches

There are many other possible combinations for lunch which is prepared by yourself but they are not appropriate to this book where we are specifically concentrating on quick and healthy solutions to maintaining a low-carb diet whilst following a hectic lifestyle. If the preparation of a packed lunch takes too much time you simply won't be able to follow the diet and it will fail. The aim is to convince you that, providing you have the will to diet (not willpower which is unnecessary on this diet) there are ways in which everyone can maintain the system, irrespective of how busy they may be in their personal life.

Salad lunchboxes

The salad lunchbox is the perfect lunch for someone
with a busy lifestyle who would prefer to make lunch
themselves. Unlike the 'standard' diet salad lunchbox
which consists of lettuce and tomato, no vinaigrettes,
mayonnaise or sauces, and a little dry meat or poultry
– which is certainly neither appetising nor effective –
this is completely different. Firstly you can have as
much low-carb food (pages 35 and 37–38) as you like,
so there is no question of hunger or irritability, and
secondly you can include tasty vinaigrette or
mayonnaise which is absolutely essential both to satisfy
your appetite and taste-buds! All you need is a standard
plastic lunchbox *with a good seal*, disposable cutlery and
a paper napkin. Remember to carry the lunchbox in an
upright position – not on its side – if you don't want to
survey a disaster for lunch. Seems obvious, but it's an
easy mistake to make. The meal tastes the same but
does not have the same aesthetic appeal!

Buy a package of salad of your choice once per week
at the supermarket; there is a wide selection available,
for example mixed crispy salad leaves, mixed watercress
and rocket or simply baby spinach leaves. A package of
salad leaves is much more convenient than purchasing
individual ingredients and mixing them yourself, which
almost always involves boredom (as you have to
consume the entire lettuce(s) within a few days) and
wastage. With some mayonnaise and a selection of
vinaigrettes you have the basis of an immense variety of
possible lunches. Here are some suggestions, but, as we
are sure you can now appreciate, the choices in low-carb
dieting are virtually unlimited. You don't have to stick
rigidly to the quantities in the following suggestions
because the ingredients are all very low-carb so larger
servings will not ruin your diet. Hunger is the cause of

most diets failing because it leads to the carbohydrate 'quick fix' of biscuits, chocolate or cakes. There is no possible need for hunger on this diet and, in fact, you are positively encouraged never to allow yourself to be hungry. Of course, the contents of lunch boxes can be simple or complicated according to your taste, but the following have all been selected on the basis of speed of preparation (as well as nutrition and low-carb content). All of the salad leaves are pre-packaged from supermarkets.

You can prepare a salad lunchbox the previous evening but it is tastier if prepared in the morning. The salad will undoubtedly be rather limp and 'soggy' the next day if you have added vinaigrette, so definitely don't add the vinaigrette until the last moment. But this small requirement should present no obstacle to enjoying these meals even to the most hectic household in the morning.

One of the most obvious differences between salad lunchboxes and sandwiches – even open sandwiches – is the carbohydrate content per serving. When you remove the bread completely (in the lunchbox) the carbohydrate content of delicious healthy meals assumes almost insignificant proportions.

Chicken breast with chilli sauce

If you decide to cook the chicken breast rather than purchase ready-cooked, remember to cook the chicken *the previous evening*. Realistically, there will not be time in the morning to cook chicken, so with a little (and we mean *very* little) preparation the previous evening, you can enjoy a delicious (and relatively inexpensive) lunch-on-the-run.

For 1
1 chicken breast
25 grams unsalted butter, cubed
½ Lebanese cucumber, cubed

4 cherry tomatoes on-the-vine, halved
2 tsp chilli sauce
30 grams (approximately) rocket and watercress leaves
freshly ground black pepper

- Place the chicken breast in an oven-safe dish and dot with cubes of butter.
- Cover with pierced aluminium foil and cook in the centre of a pre-heated oven at 180°C (gas 4) for 35–40 minutes, then set aside to cool.

Or
- Purchase a ready-cooked chicken breast.

- Slice the chicken breast and mix the chicken with the cucumber, tomatoes and chilli sauce in a medium bowl.
- Lay a bed of rocket and watercress leaves in the base of the lunchbox and top with the chilli chicken mixture.
- Season to taste with freshly ground black pepper.

CARBOHYDRATE CONTENT PER SERVING: 4 GRAMS

Egg mayonnaise with fresh basil and chives

Meals with mayonnaise appear in several parts of the book, not because we are trying to encourage this meal in your diet, but rather because mayonnaise slows the absorption of foods, satisfying hunger for longer and removing the temptation to snack between meals.

For 1
1 large free-range egg
2 tsp mayonnaise
1 tsp chopped fresh basil
1 tsp chopped fresh chives

30 grams (approximately) baby spinach leaves
pinch of paprika

- Hard boil the egg for 6–8 minutes.
- Chop the egg finely and mix with the mayonnaise, basil and chives in a medium bowl.
- Lay a bed of baby spinach leaves in the base of the lunchbox and top with the egg mayonnaise mixture.
- Garnish with a pinch of paprika.

CARBOHYDRATE CONTENT PER SERVING: 1 GRAM

Roast ham with Leerdammer cheese and mustard

For 1

30 grams (approximately) red lettuce salad leaves (radiccio, red oak lettuce, lollo rosso) – available from supermarkets
drizzle French vinaigrette
2–3 slices thick honey-roast ham (from delis or supermarkets)
1 slice Leerdammer cheese (pre-sliced from supermarket)
1 tsp wholegrain mustard
freshly ground black pepper

- Lay a bed of red lettuce salad in the lunchbox.
- Drizzle over a little French vinaigrette. This can be easily home-made (page 273) and stored for later use, or commercial.
- Top with the honey-roast ham and Leerdammer cheese, with 1 tsp of delicious wholegrain mustard.
- Season to taste with freshly ground black pepper.

CARBOHYDRATE CONTENT PER SERVING: 1 GRAM

Avocado with Bocconcini cheese

The peppery flavour of the wild rocket complements the balsamic avocado.

For 1
½ medium, ripe Hass avocado, peeled, stone
  removed, diced
50 grams (approximately) Bocconcini cheese, cubed
3 small plum tomatoes on-the-vine, quartered
2 spring onions, finely chopped
drizzle balsamic vinegar
30 grams (approximately) wild rocket leaves
freshly ground black pepper

- Mix together the avocado, Bocconcini, tomatoes and
  spring onions in a medium bowl and drizzle over
  some balsamic vinegar.
- Lay a bed of wild rocket leaves in the lunchbox and
  top with the balsamic avocado mixture.
- Season to taste with freshly ground black pepper.

CARBOHYDRATE CONTENT PER SERVING: 4 GRAMS

Tuna mayonnaise with basil and coriander

For 1
200 gram tin tuna (in brine), drained and flaked
1 tbsp mayonnaise
2 tsp chopped fresh basil
2 tsp chopped fresh coriander
1 spring onion, finely chopped
30 grams (approximately) fresh watercress
freshly ground black pepper

- Mix together the tuna, mayonnaise, basil, coriander,
  and spring onion in a medium bowl.
- Lay a bed of watercress in the base of the lunchbox
  and top with the tuna mixture.

• Season to taste with freshly ground black pepper.

CARBOHYDRATE CONTENT PER SERVING: 1 GRAM

Roast beef and pickle

Although commercially-prepared pickles have a reasonably high carbohydrate content (approximately 35 grams per hundred grams), as you only use about 2 teaspoons per meal, this equates to only 3–4 grams of carbohydrate per meal which is almost insignificant.

For 1
30 grams (approximately) crispy green lettuce (green oak, frisée, coral, mizuna)
drizzle of French vinaigrette
2–3 slices roast beef (available from delis or supermarkets)
2–3 medium pickled onions, drained
1 tsp Branston pickle
50 grams Cheddar cheese, cubed

• Lay a bed of crispy green lettuce leaves in the base of the lunchbox.
• Drizzle over some French vinaigrette, to taste.
• Place the slices of roast beef on the salad, and top with pickled onions, Branston pickle and Cheddar cheese.

CARBOHYDRATE CONTENT PER SERVING: 4 GRAMS

Salmon with crème fraîche

For 1
1 medium salmon fillet, approximately 125–150 grams
30 grams unsalted butter, cubed
¼ Lebanese cucumber, diced
1 tsp chopped fresh chives
75 ml crème fraîche

147

30 grams (approximately) wild rocket leaves
drizzle of French vinaigrette
2 small plum tomatoes on-the-vine, halved
freshly ground black pepper

- Place the salmon fillet in a shallow oven-safe dish, dot with butter, cover with pierced aluminium foil and cook in the centre of a pre-heated oven at 180°C (gas 4) for 12–15 minutes.

Or
- Place the salmon fillet in a microwave-safe dish, pour over a tablespoon of water, cover and cook on 'high' for 2½ minutes, then allow to stand for a further minute.

At the same time
- Mix together the cucumber, chives and crème fraîche in a small bowl.
- Lay a bed of wild rocket leaves in the base of the lunchbox and drizzle over some French vinaigrette.
- Place the salmon fillet on the rocket.
- Arrange the tomatoes around the salmon and spoon the cucumber crème fraîche onto the salmon.
- Season to taste with freshly ground black pepper.

CARBOHYDRATE CONTENT PER SERVING: 4 GRAMS

Greek salad

For 1
¼ cucumber, diced
4 cherry tomatoes on-the-vine, halved
2 spring onions, finely chopped
25 grams feta cheese, cubed
25 grams Halloumi cheese, cubed
3 green olives
3 black olives

30 grams (approximately) mixed green salad leaves
  (coral, green oak leaf, curly endive, cos)
drizzle of French vinaigrette
freshly ground black pepper

- Mix together the cucumber, tomatoes, spring onions,
  cubed cheese, olives and mixed salad leaves.
- Drizzle over a little French vinaigrette and season to
  taste with freshly ground black pepper.

CARBOHYDRATE CONTENT PER SERVING: 3 GRAMS

Chicken with curry and herb sauce

The recipe for the sauce is very quick and easy but
you can substitute commercial curry sauce if you
prefer, providing it is a low-carb curry sauce.

For 1
1 chicken breast
30 grams rocket leaves
3 cherry tomatoes on-the-vine
1 spring onion, finely chopped
pinch of Cayenne pepper

Curry and herb sauce
2 tbsp soured cream
2 tbsp mayonnaise
2 tsp medium curry powder
1 tsp tomato ketchup
1 tsp chopped fresh coriander
1 tsp chopped fresh basil

- Cook the chicken breast (the evening before use)
  according to the method described on pages 63–64.

Or
- Purchase a ready-cooked chicken breast.

149

- Chop the chicken breast into medium cubes.
- Mix together the ingredients of the curry and herb sauce in a medium bowl, then stir in the cooked chicken breast.
- Lay a bed of rocket leaves in the base of the lunchbox, top with chicken in curry and herb sauce, and dot with cherry tomatoes.
- Sprinkle over the finely chopped spring onions and Cayenne pepper, to garnish.

CARBOHYDRATE CONTENT PER SERVING: 4 GRAMS

Tiger prawns with chilli and coriander vinaigrette

This is so simple to prepare, providing you plan to have the ingredients available, and so delicious. We would strongly advise you to make your own vinaigrette rather than buy a commercial variety. It takes moments to make, is *much* less expensive, and can be adapted in many different ways. Of course a commercial vinaigrette is just as effective – but always remember to check the carbohydrate content as it can vary from virtually zero to unacceptable levels! The vinaigrettes to avoid are the 'low-fat' variety as they are usually higher in carbohydrate content.

For 1
1 tsp chopped fresh coriander
¼ green chilli, deseeded and finely diced
2 tbsp French vinaigrette, home-made (page 273) or commercial
8 pre-cooked tiger prawns, shelled
1 small yellow pepper, deseeded and diced
30 grams (approximately) watercress and rocket salad leaves
freshly ground black pepper

- Mix together the coriander, chilli and vinaigrette in a medium bowl.
- Stir in the tiger prawns and diced yellow pepper and marinate for at least 20 minutes (preferably overnight). If you don't have any time in the morning omit the marinating period.
- Place the watercress and rocket leaves in the base of the lunchbox and top up with the tiger prawns in chilli and coriander vinaigrette.
- Season to taste with freshly ground black pepper.

CARBOHYDRATE CONTENT PER SERVING: 3 GRAMS

Tiger prawns with lemon and coriander vinaigrette

If you don't like chilli in the above recipe, simply omit the chilli and substitute 1 tablespoon of freshly squeezed lemon juice for a delicious lemon and coriander vinaigrette.

CARBOHYDRATE CONTENT PER SERVING: 3 GRAMS

Port Salut, courgettes and chives salad

For 1
2 medium courgettes, thinly sliced
50 grams Port Salut cheese, sliced
4 small plum vine tomatoes, quartered lengthways
1 spring onion, finely chopped
30 grams (approximately) crispy herb salad (green oak, frisée, mizuna with basil and coriander leaves)
drizzle of balsamic vinaigrette
freshly ground black pepper

- Mix together the courgettes, Port Salut cheese, tomatoes and spring onion with the herb salad

151

leaves and drizzle over the balsamic vinaigrette.
• Season to taste with freshly ground black pepper.

CARBOHYDRATE CONTENT PER SERVING: 4 GRAMS

Of course, any of the multitude of low-carb suggested fillings for open sandwiches are equally suitable for a salad lunchbox, such as:

Tuna pâté
Tiger prawns with mayonnaise
Chicken tikka
Bacon and tomato
Prawn mayonnaise
Duck à l'orange pâté
Chicken salad
Chicken, salsa and avocado
Steak salad
Egg and cress
Chicken and bacon
Cheese (of multiple varieties) and pickles
Smoked ham and mustard
Salmon and cucumber
Roasted peppers and sun-dried tomatoes
Roast beef and horseradish sauce
Cheese and celery with mayonnaise
Salmon with mayonnaise
Guacamole
Egg and prawns
Avocado, mozzarella and sun-dried tomatoes
Roast pork with apple sauce
Smoked turkey breast with cranberry sauce
Emmental cheese with crispy pancetta
Chargrilled peppers with chicken
Bacon, lettuce and tomato
Avocado with tomato and mayonnaise
Coronation chicken with green salad
Pastrami with wholegrain mustard and pickled onions

Sandwiches

Two slices of bread at lunchtime is the equivalent of
30–34 grams of carbohydrate which is simply too much
for a successful low-carb diet. There are two possible
solutions, both of which are equally successful in
solving the problem.

- As previously described, discard the upper layer of
  bread when you intend to consume the meal and
  enjoy a very satisfying and nutritious open
  sandwich – without the excess carbohydrates.
- An easier solution is to *carry the sandwich as an
  open sandwich*. At first glance this would seem
  impossible: how can you possibly transport an open
  sandwich? Actually it is very simple! Many
  manufacturers (e.g. Lakeland) market a plastic
  container designed to carry a large sandwich. It has
  a rectangular shape which is the perfect size and
  shape to seal in the sandwich, but not to allow the
  sandwich to move within the container (which
  happens with a normal rectangular sealed plastic
  container). This is ideal for transporting an open
  sandwich. Simply place the lower half of the
  sandwich in the base of the container, top with a
  large low-carb filling of choice and seal the
  container. This will transport your open sandwich
  simply and cleanly, ready for you to enjoy at your
  convenience. Open sandwiches can be notoriously
  difficult to consume gracefully – especially if
  packed with lots of delicious filling – so disposable
  cutlery and a napkin are definitely advisable!

Carbohydrates in the form of bread (or bread products)
are just a mode of transporting food. They add very
little to the taste – and virtually nothing to the
nutrition – so any method to reduce your intake of
carbohydrates has to be beneficial to your health.

Carbohydrates are just 'fillers' in any meal. They fill you up (usually with uncomfortable abdominal distension), cause lethargy and stimulate insulin production which leads to further hypoglycaemia and all the inevitable sequelae: irritability, tremor, poor concentration and the need for another carbohydrate 'quick fix'. Refined carbohydrates simply are not good for your health and you do not need them.

On a low-carb diet the sandwich fillings are really only limited by your personal preferences and appetite! Almost all sandwich fillings are naturally low-carb; the bread is the problem. Adhere to the guidelines on pages 107–10 and you will diet successfully. Obviously all of the take-away sandwiches described on pages 125–27 can equally successfully be included in a lunch made at home – and much more economically. Simply remember to purchase a selection of cold meats, poultry, fish, cheeses, sauces or vinaigrettes and salad on your weekly shopping list and you will be prepared for lunch for the entire week.

A single package of mixed watercress, rocket and spinach leaves will form the basis of many sandwiches. Pre-packaged sliced cold meats or poultry can last for days; even smoked salmon is very economical by this method as it can be purchased in very small quantities (in sealed packages) and, mixed with mayonnaise and chopped fresh herbs, will last for several meals. All the sandwiches from a take-away (pages 125–27) and all the menu suggestions from the deli (pages 127–29) can be easily purchased in advance from the supermarket and incorporated in your packed lunch.

Here are some additional suggestions for suitably delicious and healthy sandwiches in your low-carb lifestyle. All the following sandwiches are described with two slices of bread (the upper layer of which would have to be discarded, as described). Of course, all can equally (and more successfully for your diet) be created as open sandwiches with the lower half of a bread roll and the designated container (described above) for a more effective low-carb diet.

Chicken with mayonnaise and avocado open sandwich

For 2

1 small chicken breast fillet
2 tbsp extra-virgin olive oil
1 tbsp mayonnaise
2 slices buttered wholemeal bread
½ a small ripe Hass avocado, peeled, stone removed, finely sliced
freshly ground black pepper

- Sauté the chicken fillet in the olive oil for approximately 5 minutes on each side, turning once.
- Set aside to cool, then slice finely.
- Mix with the mayonnaise and spoon onto a slice of buttered wholemeal bread.
- Arrange the avocado slices on the chicken and season to taste with freshly ground black pepper

CARBOHYDRATE CONTENT PER SERVING: 19 GRAMS
(ONLY 2 GRAMS WITHOUT BREAD)

Ham, egg and chives open sandwich

For 2

2 thick slices pre-cooked honey-roast ham
2 slices buttered wholemeal bread
I hard-boiled egg, sliced
2 medium plum tomatoes, thinly sliced
drizzle of Balsamic vinaigrette
1 tbsp fresh chives, snipped
freshly ground black pepper

- Lay the slices of honey-roast ham on the bread.
- Top with slices of egg and tomato, and drizzle over Balsamic vinaigrette, to taste.
- Sprinkle with chopped chives, and season to taste with freshly ground black pepper.

CARBOHYDRATE CONTENT PER SERVING: 19 GRAMS

(ONLY 2 GRAMS WITHOUT BREAD)

Prawn mayonnaise open sandwich

For 2

150 grams cooked prawns
1 tbsp mayonnaise
2 spring onions, finely chopped
2 slices buttered wholemeal bread
freshly ground black pepper

- Mix together the prawns, mayonnaise and chopped spring onions.
- Spoon the mixture on two slices of buttered wholemeal bread.
- Season to taste with freshly ground black pepper.

CARBOHYDRATE CONTENT PER SERVING: 18 GRAMS

(1 GRAM WITHOUT BREAD)

Tuna mayonnaise open sandwich

We suggest using tuna in brine or springwater – not to avoid the oil – but because tuna in brine is easily drained and can then absorb the flavours of mayonnaise and other additives more easily.

For 2

200 gram tin tuna (in brine or springwater), drained
1 tbsp mayonnaise
1 tbsp chopped fresh basil
1 tsp chopped fresh coriander

freshly ground black pepper
2 slices buttered wholemeal bread
1 vine-ripened tomato, diced (optional)
½ small red pepper, deseeded and sliced thinly
(optional)
1 tsp chopped fresh chives

- Flake the tuna and mix with 1 tbsp mayonnaise,
chopped basil and coriander, and freshly ground
black pepper.
- Spoon the mixture liberally on two slices of
buttered wholemeal bread.
- Top with diced vine-ripened tomato (and/or sliced
red pepper with chopped fresh chives).

CARBOHYDRATE CONTENT PER SERVING: 19 GRAMS
(2 GRAMS WITHOUT BREAD)

Bacon, lettuce and tomato open sandwich

A classic sandwich, which is easily converted for use in
the low-carb diet by discarding the upper slice of bread.

For 2
4 rashers cooked bacon
small handful of mixed lettuce leaves (frisée, mizuna,
green oak, rocket)
2 slices buttered wholemeal bread (or toast)
2 medium plum tomatoes (preferably on-the-vine),
sliced
drizzle of Worcestershire sauce, to taste
freshly ground black pepper

- Cook the bacon, either fry, grill or by microwave
(pages 91–92).
- Arrange the mixed lettuce leaves on the buttered
wholemeal bread (or toast, if preferred).
- Top with tomato slices and cooked bacon rashers.

- Drizzle over a few drops of Worcestershire sauce (optional) and season to taste with freshly ground black pepper.

CARBOHYDRATE CONTENT PER SERVING: 19 GRAMS
(ONLY 2 GRAMS WITHOUT BREAD)

Crab salad open sandwich

For 2

200 grams white crab meat (tinned or fresh)
1 tbsp mayonnaise
1 tbsp chopped fresh basil
½ small Hass avocado, peeled, stone removed, finely sliced
1 large plum tomato, diced
2 slices buttered wholemeal bread
freshly ground black pepper

- Mix together the crab meat, mayonnaise, basil, avocado and tomato in a medium bowl.
- Spread on two slices of buttered wholemeal bread and season to taste.

CARBOHYDRATE CONTENT PER SERVING: 19 GRAMS
(2 GRAMS WITHOUT BREAD!)

Salsa steak open sandwich

For 2

2 tbsp extra-virgin olive oil
200 grams minute steak
2 slices buttered wholemeal bread
50 grams of salsa
freshly ground black pepper

- Heat the olive oil in a medium frying pan.
- Fry the minute steak for 2 minutes per side.

- Place on buttered wholemeal bread and top with prepared salsa.
- Season to taste with freshly ground black pepper and serve immediately.

CARBOHYDRATE CONTENT PER SERVING: 20 GRAMS
(ONLY 3 GRAMS WITHOUT BREAD)

Salami salad open sandwich

The problem of having such a wide availability of choice in various foods is that there is also a wide variability in their contents. Individual salamis may vary from virtually no carbohydrate content (the ultimate) to a significant carbohydrate content so you have to check the label (if purchased from a supermarket). Deli salamis are almost all low in carbohydrates.

For 2
6 slices salami (of choice), chopped
1 medium plum tomato, finely sliced
50 grams Emmental cheese, grated
1 tbsp chopped fresh parsley (optional)
1 tbsp mayonnaise
freshly ground black pepper
2 slices buttered wholemeal bread

- Mix together the salami, tomato, cheese, parsley and mayonnaise in a medium bowl.
- Season with freshly ground black pepper.
- Spread on two slices buttered wholemeal bread.

CARBOHYDRATE CONTENT PER SERVING: 19 GRAMS
(2 GRAMS WITHOUT BREAD)

Lunch at home

Lunch at home can be either a simple open sandwich, a light salad or a lightly cooked meal. As you can appreciate there is considerable overlap between the various chapters as many light meals are just as applicable to breakfast, lunch or supper. The pace of modern life has removed the rigid protocol which once directed our eating habits. The recipes described have features in common: all are made from healthy ingredients which are low in carbohydrates, readily available and relatively quickly prepared. For light lunches which take a little longer to prepare we would suggest you consult *The New High Protein Diet* and *The New High Protein Diet Cookbook*, published by Vermilion.

Here are a selection of light, quick-and-easy low-carb lunches which would be equally suitable for light supper.

Hot-and-spicy chicken drumsticks with baby spinach leaves

Pre-cooked chicken drumsticks are widely available from supermarkets and Marks and Spencer. They are available either plain or coated with a variety of sauces: barbecue, tikka, Chinese and tandoori. However if you have the time available, or would prefer to cook them yourself, the method and the recipe for the sauce is described below. The carbohydrate content is about the same for both methods of preparation.

For 2
2 medium plum tomatoes on-the-vine, chopped
1 medium Lebanese cucumber, chopped
2 spring onions, finely chopped
1 tbsp mayonnaise
100 grams pre-washed baby spinach leaves
pinch of paprika

freshly ground black pepper

4 pre-cooked chicken drumsticks coated with hot and spicy sauce

- Mix together the tomatoes, cucumber and spring onions with the mayonnaise.
- Place a bed of baby spinach leaves in the centre of each plate and spoon the mayonnaise mixture onto the spinach.
- Sprinkle over a little paprika and season to taste with freshly ground black pepper.
- Add the pre-cooked drumsticks, and enjoy.

Alternatively, if you have time (or prefer) to cook the drumsticks yourself you will need:

4 chicken drumsticks, skin on, scored diagonally on each side

2 tbsp extra-virgin olive oil

Marinade

2 tbsp light soy sauce

2 tbsp sweet sherry

1 garlic clove, peeled and grated

2 slices fresh root ginger, peeled and finely chopped

3–4 drops Tabasco sauce

- Mix the soy sauce, sherry, garlic, ginger and Tabasco sauce in a medium bowl, add the drumsticks and marinate for 3–4 hours.
- Brush the drumsticks with extra-virgin olive oil, and barbecue (or grill) for about 10–12 minutes, turning regularly and basting with the marinade.

CARBOHYDRATE CONTENT PER SERVING: 6 GRAMS
(WITH PREPARED DRUMSTICKS),
4 GRAMS (WITH HOME-MADE DRUMSTICKS AND MARINADE)

Haddock with herbs

Obviously this recipe is best with fresh fish but it's not always possible to obtain fresh fish. The solution is simple: buy fresh fish (either from the fishmonger or supermarket) and freeze for later use, or buy frozen fish fillets (without batter or dressing). Thawing by microwave takes a very short time and means that you can enjoy fish at any time, irrespective of how busy your schedule.

For 2
2 medium haddock fillets
2 shallots, peeled and finely chopped
1 tbsp chopped fresh flat-leaf parsley
1 tbsp chopped fresh coriander
2 slices fresh root ginger, peeled and finely chopped
100 ml dry white wine
freshly ground black pepper
sprigs of fresh dill, to garnish

- Place the haddock fillets in an oven-safe dish and top with the shallots, parsley, coriander and ginger.
- Pour the wine over the fish, cover with pierced aluminium foil and cook in the centre of a pre-heated oven at 180°C (gas 4) for 15–18 minutes.
- Season to taste and serve immediately, garnished with sprigs of fresh dill.

Quick method
- Place the haddock fillets in a microwave-safe dish and top with the shallots, parsley, coriander and ginger.
- Pour 2 tablespoons wine over the fish, cover with the appropriate cover for the container (not aluminium foil!) and cook in the centre of a

microwave oven (850W) for 2½ minutes. Increase the time by a third (to about 3 minutes) for a 650–750W oven.

- Season to taste and serve immediately, garnished with sprigs of fresh dill.

CARBOHYDRATE CONTENT PER SERVING: 2 GRAMS

Gammon steaks with balsamic vinegar

Gammon is a rich source of all essential amino acids and many vitamins, especially vitamin B_1.

For 2
2 tbsp extra-virgin olive oil
2 unsmoked gammon steaks (about 150 grams each)
2 tbsp balsamic vinegar
freshly ground black pepper
crispy herb salad (page 263)

- Heat the extra-virgin olive oil in a large frying pan and fry the gammon steaks for about 4 minutes, turning once.
- Pour the balsamic vinegar over the gammon steaks and cook for a further minute.
- Season to taste with freshly ground black pepper and serve immediately with a crispy herb salad.

CARBOHYDRATE CONTENT PER SERVING: 7 GRAMS

Smoked trout with avocado

Smoked trout is relatively inexpensive as you only need a small amount because the 'richness' of the meal is very satisfying. You simply cannot overindulge on food of this quality because it naturally satisfies the appetite.

For 2

1 large avocado, peeled, stone removed, thinly sliced
juice of a freshly squeezed lemon
200 grams smoked trout, sliced
2 spring onions, finely chopped
1 tbsp chopped fresh dill
1 tbsp crème fraîche
freshly ground black pepper
pinch of paprika

- Arrange the slices of avocado as a fan on two plates.
- Sprinkle over the lemon juice (for flavour and to prevent discolouration of the avocado).
- Mix together the smoked trout, spring onions, dill and crème fraîche in a medium bowl and season to taste.
- Spoon the mixture into the centre of the avocado fan, season and garnish with a pinch of paprika.

CARBOHYDRATE CONTENT PER SERVING: 4 GRAMS

Spicy prawns with rocket

Shellfish are a particularly rich source of the mineral zinc which is essential for the production of insulin.

For 2

150 grams cooked prawns, rinsed
100 grams wild rocket leaves, washed
freshly ground black pepper
1 spring onion, finely chopped, to garnish (optional)

Spicy mayonnaise

1 tbsp mayonnaise
2 tsp medium-strength curry powder
  (or 'hot' if you prefer)
1 tsp tomato sauce

- Mix together the mayonnaise, curry powder and tomato sauce in a small bowl and stir in the prawns.
- Lay the wild rocket leaves in the centre of each plate and spoon over the spicy prawn mixture.
- Season to taste and sprinkle over the finely chopped spring onion.

CARBOHYDRATE CONTENT PER SERVING: 2 GRAMS

Tandoori lamb with cucumber raita

For 2
1 tbsp tandoori paste
150 ml natural yoghurt
2 large lamb chops (approximately 125–150 grams each)
cucumber raita (page 276)
75 grams watercress
freshly ground black pepper

- Mix together the tandoori paste and natural yoghurt and coat the lamb chops with the mixture.
- Grill the lamb chops under a hot grill, no closer than 8–10 cm from the grill, for about 8 minutes, turning once.

At the same time
- Prepare the cucumber raita.
- Serve the tandoori lamb with the cucumber raita and watercress and season to taste.

CARBOHYDRATE CONTENT PER SERVING: 14 GRAMS

Tuna with spinach and basil

This delicious meal is equally suitable as a light supper. Tuna is a rich source of essential omega-3 fatty acids and spinach provides vitamin C and the element iron.

For 2
50 grams unsalted butter
100 grams spinach leaves
6 cherry tomatoes, halved
1 tbsp chopped fresh basil
185 gram tin tuna (in brine), drained
1 tbsp mayonnaise
2 spring onions, finely chopped
freshly ground black pepper

- Heat the butter in a medium frying pan (or wok) and lightly sauté the spinach, cherry tomatoes and ½ tablespoon chopped basil for 1–2 minutes (or until the spinach softens), stirring frequently. Be careful not to overcook!

At the same time
- Mix together the tuna, mayonnaise, chopped spring onions and remaining ½ tablespoon of chopped basil in a medium bowl.
- Spoon the spinach mixture onto the centre of each two plates and top with the tuna mayonnaise.
- Season to taste.

This meal can also be enjoyed as a cold salad. Simply mix together the spinach, cherry tomatoes and basil, place in the centre of two plates and top with tuna mayonnaise.

CARBOHYDRATE CONTENT PER SERVING: 4 GRAMS

Savoury crêpes

Savoury crêpes are perfect for light lunch, supper or even breakfast! As each crêpe contains only 5–6 grams of carbohydrate (or about one third of the amount of carbohydrate in a single slice of bread) you can enjoy crêpes in moderation as the crêpe itself is only a transport medium for the filling, and you can be as adventurous as you want in designer, quickly-prepared, low-carb fillings. This recipe can be made by hand or using a blender.

For 2
50 grams plain flour
pinch of salt
1 large free-range egg, beaten
150 ml full-cream milk
1 tbsp melted butter

- Sieve the flour and salt into a medium bowl.
- Add ½ of the beaten egg mixture, whisking constantly.
- Gradually blend in the milk, drawing the mixture to the centre of the bowl until you achieve an even consistency.
- Allow to stand for at least ½ hour before making the crêpes.
- Just before cooking, stir the melted butter into the mixture.

Crêpes can be made by either the traditional method or by using a commercial crêpe-maker. Commercial crêpe-makers are not expensive and effectively allow crêpes to be included as an integral part of a quick low-carb diet.

Traditional method
- Add a level tablespoon of butter to a small non-stick frying pan, melt the butter over medium heat and evenly coat the pan.
- Add 2 tablespoons of the mixture to the pan, then tip the pan to evenly coat the base of the pan. Cook for about 20–30 seconds and remove with a pallete knife.

Crêpe-maker
- Pour the mixture into a wide shallow dish.
- Turn on the crêpe-maker. When hot, dip the crêpe-maker horizonally onto the mixture to lightly coat and allow the crêpe to cook. When the edge of the crêpe is lightly browned, remove with a pallete spatula and repeat the process.

Savoury crêpes can either be rolled around the selected filling, folded in half over the filling or folded into triangles and topped with the savoury filling. Here are some suggestions for lunch savoury crêpes which are equally suitable for light supper.

Hoisin duck crêpes

For 2
6 crêpes (as above)
3 tbsp extra-virgin olive oil
250 grams duck breast, sliced into strips
6 spring onions, halved lengthways
3 slices fresh root ginger, peeled and sliced julienne
2 tbsp hoisin sauce
30 ml chicken stock
1 tbsp chopped fresh basil
freshly ground black pepper

- Prepare the crêpes (pages 166–68).
- Heat the extra-virgin olive oil in a wok and stir-fry the duck breast for 3–4 minutes.
- Add the spring onions, ginger, hoisin sauce and chicken stock to the wok and stir-fry for 2–3 minutes, then add the basil and stir-fry for a final 2 minutes.
- Season to taste and spoon immediately onto the crêpes, then fold the crêpes in half.

CARBOHYDRATE CONTENT PER SERVING (3 CRÊPES): 24 GRAMS

Prawn mayonnaise crêpes

For 2
6 crêpes
100 grams pre-cooked prawns
1 tbsp mayonnaise
½ tbsp chopped fresh coriander
½ tbsp chopped fresh chives
pinch of Cayenne pepper

- Prepare the crêpes (pages 166–68).

At the same time
- Mix together the prawns, mayonnaise, coriander and chives.
- Stir in a pinch of Cayenne pepper.
- Spoon the mixture evenly over the crêpes, then fold the crêpes in half, and serve immediately.

CARBOHYDRATE CONTENT PER SERVING (3 CRÊPES): 15 GRAMS

Spinach and Emmental crêpes

For 2
6 crêpes
15 grams unsalted butter
15 grams plain flour
150 ml full-cream milk
100 grams Emmental cheese, grated
75 grams spinach leaves
1 tbsp chopped fresh flat-leaf parsley
freshly ground black pepper

- Prepare the crêpes (pages 166–67).
- Melt the butter in a medium saucepan, remove from the heat and stir in the flour.
- Return to a low heat and gradually blend in the milk.
- When the sauce begins to thicken, stir in the grated Emmental cheese.
- Season to taste.

At the same time

- Lightly steam (or microwave) the spinach for 3–4 minutes.
- Chop the spinach leaves and mix with the chopped parsley.

- Mix the spinach and parsley into the cheese sauce. Spoon the mixture evenly over the crêpes, then fold the crêpes in half.
- Serve immediately.

CARBOHYDRATE CONTENT PER SERVING (3 CRÊPES): 26 GRAMS

Cod with orange sauce

Cod and orange complement one another nutritionally, with essential amino acids and B vitamins from cod and vitamin C from the orange.

For 2
2 medium cod fillets
1 large free-range egg, beaten
1 tbsp plain flour (optional)
3 tbsp extra-virgin olive oil
juice of a freshly squeezed large orange
75 ml crème fraîche
75 grams watercress
freshly ground black pepper

- Coat the cod fillets in egg then plain flour.
- Heat the extra-virgin olive oil in a medium frying pan and cook the cod for 4–5 minutes, turning once.

At the same time
- Mix together the orange juice and crème fraîche, then pour into a small saucepan and heat through gently. Do not boil!

- Serve the cod with watercress, add the sauce and season to taste.

CARBOHYDRATE CONTENT PER SERVING: 11 GRAMS
(5 GRAMS IF FLOUR IS OMITTED)

Steak with asparagus purée

For 2

200 grams asparagus (approximately 10 spears),
  washed and trimmed
½ tbsp chopped fresh basil
½ tbsp chopped fresh coriander
1 tbsp freshly squeezed lemon juice
2 tbsp extra-virgin olive oil
250 grams minute steak
radicchio and cucumber salad (page 267)
freshly ground black pepper

- Place the asparagus in the base of a suitable microwave-safe container, arranging the thick stalks to the outside of the dish and the thin tops facing inwards.
- Add 2 tbsp water, cover and cook on 'high' for 2–3 minutes, then allow to stand for 1 minute.

Or
- Lightly steam the asparagus for 10-12 minutes.

- Transfer the asparagus to a blender, add the basil, coriander and lemon juice and purée.

At the same time
- Heat the extra-virgin olive oil in a medium frying pan and fry the steak for 4–5 minutes, turning once. The steak can be grilled for the same length of time, if preferred.

And
- Prepare the radicchio and cucumber salad.
- Transfer the steak to warm plates, top with asparagus purée, season to taste and serve with radicchio and cucumber salad.

CARBOHYDRATE CONTENT PER SERVING: 11 GRAMS

Chargrilled Madras sardines with crème fraîche

Sardines are one of the healthiest foods available, providing a rich source of essential omega-3 fatty acids, vitamin D and calcium.

For 2
2 x 120 gram tins sardines in oil, drained
2 tbsp Madras curry paste (or medium, according to preference)
1 tbsp chopped fresh coriander
4 tbsp crème fraîche
1 tsp turmeric

- Coat the sardines with the curry paste.
- Line a grill tray with aluminium foil, then lay the sardines in a single layer on the grill tray.
- Grill under a hot grill (no closer than 8–10 cm from the grill) for 2–3 minutes, turning once.

At the same time
- Mix together the crème fraîche and turmeric.

- Serve the curried sardines with the turmeric crème fraîche and garnish with chopped fresh coriander.

CARBOHYDRATE CONTENT PER SERVING: 5 GRAMS

Bistro lunch

Light lunch in a bistro is very easily adapted to the low-carb lifestyle because most of the menus are actually naturally low in carbohydrates! Good, healthy food excludes refined carbohydrates, so providing you avoid breads, pasta and rice (and, of course, desserts) there is very little else that is prohibited on this diet. Even where meals have some pulses or starchy vegetables (such as potatoes or parsnips) these should be simply left on the plate! Here are some examples of typical bistro menus. All were obtained from bistros and are authentic examples of typical meals. Chinese, Indian, Thai and Italian meals are considered in the section on Dinner Restaurant menus on pages 240–48.

Entrée

All the following can be included in the diet:

   Shrimp, crab and fennel consommé

   Mixed leaf and herb salad, with aged balsamic vinegar and olive oil

   Grilled asparagus, roasted tomatoes, pecorino and rocket salad

   Rosemary and lemon-cured wild sea trout, lambs lettuce and radish salad

   Slow roasted aubergine, vine tomato and goat's cheese galette

   Escalope of pan-fried salmon with roasted vine tomatoes, baby spinach and peppercorn

The following can be included, omitting the carbohydrates:

   Medallions of citrus, marinated monkfish with roast almonds and couscous
   Advice: Leave the couscous

   Warm smoked chicken and pomegranate salad with puy lentil salsa
   Advice: Leave the lentil salsa

Main course

All the following can be included in the diet:

Beef carpaccio with white truffle pecorino

Grilled cod fillet with Shetland mussels, seaweed, and spring onions

Grilled Scottish sirloin, asparagus and thyme jus

Loin of veal with baby fennel and sprouting broccoli

Lemon-marinated leg of lamb with wood-roasted peppers and avocado salsa

Grilled sea bass, shaved fennel and roasted cherry vine tomatoes

Côte de Bœuf with roasted pak choi and capsicum

The following can be included, omitting the carbohydrates:

Corn-fed chicken, chickpea and coriander falafel, lemon and chilli yoghurt
Advice: Leave the chickpea and coriander falafel

Roasted artichokes with chilli, tomatoes and confit potato
Advice: Leave the confit potato

Tagliolini with Scottish lobster, red pepper and Swiss chard
Advice: Obviously, no pasta, no tagliolini

Warm smoked Scottish salmon, cavolo nero, parmentier potatoes and lemon oil
Advice: Simply leave the parmentier potatoes

Breast of Trelough duck, peas and broad beans and sautéed wild mushrooms
Advice: Leave the broad beans

Welsh rack of lamb, white bean purée and beetroot confit
Advice: Once again, leave the white bean purée

Whole grilled mackerel with tabbouleh
Advice: Obviously no tabbouleh, which is virtually pure carbohydrate

Dessert

Unfortunately desserts are very high in carbohydrates so all of the following are definitely excluded from the diet:

  Atlantic chocolate bomb Safron Risotto
  Cannelloni, Swiss chard and ricotta
  Crème brulée
  Selection of ice cream and sorbets
  Knickerbocker glory
  Chocolate and hazelnut torte
  Vanilla crème brulée
  Chocolate and macadamia nut brownie with vanilla
    ice cream
  Lemon tart with mascarpone ice cream
  Banana bread with syrup berries
  Mango carpaccio with coconut sorbet
  Ice creams and sorbets, brandy snap and mixed berries

Cheese board

You can enjoy the cheese board, just leave the biscuits and crackers.

Chapter 7

Dinner

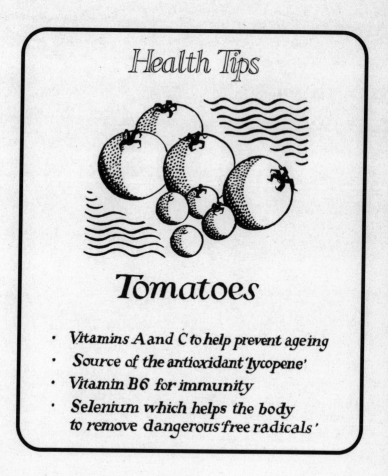

Health Tips

Tomatoes

- *Vitamins A and C to help prevent ageing*
- *Source of the antioxidant 'lycopene'*
- *Vitamin B6 for immunity*
- *Selenium which helps the body to remove dangerous 'free radicals'*

Quick-and-easy dinner at home

Salmon with lime butter sauce and
    watercress   182–83
Spicy chicken drumsticks   184
Duck with plum sauce   185
Mint cod with rocket and spinach   185–86
Chille con carne   186–87
Beef bolognaise with mushrooms   187–89
Steak with spinach and caramelised
    onions   189–90
Beef jalfrezi curry with peppers   190–91
Chicken satay with lime   192–93
Thai chicken with lemongrass and ginger   193–95
Chicken korma with mangetout and
    broccoli   195–97
Lamb tikka masala with broccoli   197–98
Turkey teriyaki   198–99
Meatballs with tomato and basil sauce   199–200
Gammon steaks with honey   200–201
Prawn omelette   201–202
Turkey in cherry tomato and chilli sauce   202–203
Thai koftas with mango raita   203–204
Turkey bolognaise with peppers   204–206
Sesame beef with ginger and lemon
    grass   206–207
Spicy scrambled eggs   207–208
Sweet and sour beef with mangetout   208–210
Gammon and aubergine with herbs   210–11
Salmon with Bocconcini and basil   211
Peking duck   212
Plaice with olives   213–14
Balti chicken   214–15
Balti pork   215
Balti beef   215
Grilled ham with mozzarella, basil and
    cherry tomatoes   215–16

Swedish meatballs with herbs   216–17
Eggs Benedict   217–18

***Really* fast suppers**
Peppered smoked ham with spinach
    and ricotta   219
Steak with cherry tomatoes, basil and
    coriander   220
Mozzarella and tomato omelette   220–21
Salmon with wild rocket and mint sauce   221–22
Pork chops with Brussels sprouts
    and citrus butter sauce   222–23
Peppered smoked mackerel with spinach
    in butter sauce   223
Bombay turkey breast with watercress
    and rocket salad   223–24
Chilli prawns   224–25
Chargrilled basil pesto salmon
    with asparagus   225–26

Dinner is usually enjoyed at home so we will consider the options for dinner under the following categories:

- Quick-and-easy dinner at home
- *Really* fast suppers
- Ready-prepared meals
- Restaurant meals

Quick-and-easy dinner at home

The essence of this book is to demonstrate how easily you can enjoy delicious, healthy meals, whether you have time to cook or not! Dinner is usually a more substantial meal than lunch, but it can still be quickly prepared using fresh ingredients or even more quickly using prepared sauces. The latter are not quite as healthy as home-made sauces, but the practical necessities of modern life dictate our lifestyle and these sauces can be essential when there simply is no time – or you're too tired – to make dinner. It's far preferable to have a healthy meal with delicious, natural ingredients and a ready-prepared sauce, than the typical pre-cooked microwave dinner.

The same message is repeated once again: the secret of successful dieting is shopping and planning ahead. You don't have to plan to the degree of a military campaign, simply keep a basic stock of ingredients always topped-up and readily available (pages 35–44). Plan your meals one day in advance and you will easily keep to the diet.

In many recipes we have provided a method using

fresh ingredients, then a quick method using prepared ingredients (like sauces), which reduces the preparation time considerably. The manufacturer of the sauces is named as these are commercial products which we have found acceptable alternatives to home-made sauces, but you certainly do not need to use these commercial varieties if you prefer other brands. In matters of commercial products it is primarily a question of personal taste. The important issue is to ensure easy compliance with your low-carb diet irrespective of how busy you are.

Once again, all the recipes include healthy ingredients and are low in carbohydrate content, but the emphasis of the recipes is primarily on speed. We have excluded many delicious recipes simply because they may take too long to prepare and therefore may not be suitable for a very busy lifestyle; for other recipes that take a little longer (and even more quick-and-easy dinner recipes) we would refer you to *The New High Protein Diet* and *The New High Protein Diet Cookbook*, both published by Vermilion.

Salmon with lime butter sauce and watercress

This recipe proves that *anyone* can cook delicious and healthy food quickly and easily – even those who think they can't cook! The meal is ready in less than 5 minutes (by microwave) and tastes delicious.

For 2
2 salmon fillets or steaks, about 150 grams each
1 lime
50 grams unsalted butter
100 grams watercress, washed
freshly ground black pepper

Microwave method

- Place the salmon fillets (or steaks) in a suitable microwave container, cover and cook on high for 2½ minutes. Allow to stand for 1 minute (no longer or they will overcook!).

At the same time
- Squeeze the lime.
- Heat the butter in a small saucepan until just melted, and add 1 tbsp of freshly squeezed lime juice.
- Heat the butter for another 30 seconds, stirring constantly.

- Serve the salmon with watercress, drizzle over the lime butter sauce and season to taste with freshly ground black pepper.

Traditional method

- Place the salmon fillets (or steaks) in an oven-safe dish, dot with butter cubes, cover with pierced aluminium foil and cook in the centre of a pre-heated oven at 180°C (gas 4) for 10–12 minutes.

At the same time
- Squeeze the lime.
- Heat the butter in a small saucepan until just melted, and add 1 tbsp of freshly squeezed lime juice.
- Heat the butter for another 30 seconds, stirring constantly.

- Serve the salmon with watercress, drizzle over the lime butter sauce and season to taste with freshly ground black pepper.

CARBOHYDRATE CONTENT PER SERVING: 2 GRAMS

Spicy chicken drumsticks

With essential amino acids and vitamins B_1, B_2 and B_3 from chicken, vitamin A from carrots and vitamin C from mangetout, this is a very healthy combination.

For 2
4 large (or 3 medium) chicken drumsticks
75 grams carrots, julienne
75 grams mangetout
freshly ground black pepper

Marinade
2 tbsp light soy sauce
2 tbsp dry sherry
1 tbsp Worcestershire sauce
1 tbsp tomato purée
2 slices fresh root ginger, peeled and finely chopped
1 garlic clove, peeled and crushed
2 tbsp extra-virgin olive oil

- Mix together the ingredients for the marinade in a medium bowl and marinate the chicken for at least 20 minutes.
- Place the chicken drumsticks on a baking tray, pour over the marinade and cook in the centre of a pre-heated oven at 180°C (gas 4) for 30–35 minutes.

Just before the drumsticks are ready
- Lightly steam (or microwave) the carrots and mangetout for 3–4 minutes.

- Season to taste and serve immediately.

CARBOHYDRATE CONTENT PER SERVING: 7 GRAMS

Duck with plum sauce

Kale is one of the richest sources of the natural antioxidant vitamin C.

For 2
3 tbsp extra-virgin olive oil
300 grams duck breast, cubed
4 shallots, peeled and chopped
1 garlic clove, peeled and chopped
3 slices fresh root ginger, peeled and chopped
75 grams button mushrooms, halved
75 grams kale, roughly chopped
1 tbsp dry sherry
2 tbsp plum sauce
50 ml chicken stock
1 tbsp chopped fresh coriander
freshly ground black pepper

- Heat the extra-virgin olive oil in a wok and stir-fry the duck breast for 3–4 minutes, then remove the duck breast from the wok with a perforated spoon and set aside.
- Add the shallots, garlic, ginger, mushrooms and kale to the wok and stir-fry for 2–3 minutes, then add the sherry, plum sauce and chicken stock.
- Return the duck breast to the wok, stir in the coriander and stir-fry for a final 3–4 minutes.
- Season to taste and serve immediately.

CARBOHYDRATE CONTENT PER SERVING: 12 GRAMS

Mint cod with rocket and spinach

Rocket is not only a rich source of vitamin C, it's also said to be a potent aphrodisiac!

For 2
3 tbsp extra-virgin olive oil
2 tbsp chopped fresh mint leaves
2 tsp freshly ground black pepper
2 medium (or large) cod fillets (about 150 grams each)
100 grams rocket and spinach leaves
lemon wedges, to garnish

- Mix together the extra-virgin olive oil, mint and black pepper in a shallow serving dish.
- Coat the cod fillets in the mixture.
- Place the fillets on a lightly-oiled baking sheet and grill under a hot grill (no closer than 8–10 cm from the grill) for 3–4 minutes, turning once.
- Serve immediately with rocket and spinach leaves, and garnish with lemon wedges.

CARBOHYDRATE CONTENT PER SERVING: 3 GRAMS

Chilli con carne

Chilli con carne is an excellent example of how a relatively high-carbohydrate meal can be easily converted into a low-carb meal; simply omit the kidney beans and serve with vegetables instead of rice! Much more nutritious (and much tastier).

For 2
2 tbsp extra-virgin olive oil
1 medium red onion, peeled and chopped
1 garlic clove, peeled and chopped
250 grams lean minced beef
1 tbsp plain flour
1 tsp chilli powder
300 ml beef stock
2 tbsp tomato purée
2 medium red peppers, deseeded and sliced
1 tbsp chopped fresh coriander leaves (optional)

freshly ground black pepper
75 grams mangetout
75 grams French beans

- Heat the extra-virgin olive oil in a large frying pan and sauté the onion and garlic for 2–3 minutes.
- Add the mince and brown for 4–5 minutes, stirring frequently.
- Remove from the heat and stir in the flour and chilli powder.
- Gradually stir in the stock and tomato purée and return to a gentle heat.
- Add the peppers and simmer gently for 10 minutes.
- Stir in the coriander (optional) and simmer for a further 5 minutes.

At the same time
- Lightly steam the mangetout and French beans for 10–12 minutes or microwave the vegetables for 3–4 minutes.
- Season to taste and serve immediately.

CARBOHYDRATE CONTENT PER SERVING: 20 GRAMS

Beef bolognaise with mushrooms

It's always important in cooking (and dieting) to realise that you don't have to follow traditional recipes. Bolognaise is a perfect example: it simply doesn't have to be served with pasta. Pasta is cheap and filling, but has no nutritional value. So try a more adventurous combination! .

For 2
2 tbsp extra-virgin olive oil
1 medium onion, peeled and diced
1 garlic clove, peeled and finely chopped
250 grams lean minced beef

2 tbsp tomato purée
200 ml beef stock
1 tbsp chopped fresh basil, or 1 tsp dried basil
  (optional)
100 grams button mushrooms, wiped and halved
100 grams sugar snap peas
freshly ground black pepper

- Heat the olive oil in a medium frying pan and sauté the onion and garlic for 1–2 minutes.
- Add the mince and brown, stirring frequently.
- Stir in the tomato purée and stock, and bring to a gentle simmer.
- Stir in the basil and mushrooms, and simmer for 5–7 minutes.

At the same time
- Lightly steam the sugar snap peas for 10–12 minutes or microwave the sugar snap peas for 3–4 minutes.
- Serve the beef bolognaise with sugar snap peas and season to taste.

CARBOHYDRATE CONTENT PER SERVING: 11 GRAMS

Quick method
If you have really no time, the following method produces even quicker results and is almost as nutritious.

For 2
2 tbsp extra-virgin olive oil
1 medium onion, peeled and diced
1 garlic clove, peeled and finely chopped
250 grams lean minced beef
320-gram jar bolognaise sauce (e.g. Dolmio)
1 tbsp chopped fresh basil, or 1 tsp dried basil
  (optional)

100 grams button mushrooms, wiped and halved
100 grams sugar snap peas
freshly ground black pepper

- Heat the olive oil in a medium frying pan and sauté the onion and garlic for 1–2 minutes.
- Add the mince and brown, stirring frequently.
- Stir in the prepared bolognaise sauce and bring to a gentle simmer.
- Stir in the basil and mushrooms, and simmer for 5–7 minutes.

At the same time
- Lightly steam the sugar snap peas for 10–12 minutes or microwave the sugar snap peas for 3–4 minutes.
- Serve the beef bolognaise with sugar snap peas and season to taste.

CARBOHYDRATE CONTENT PER SERVING: 19 GRAMS

Steak with spinach and caramelised onions

The perfect combination for an iron-rich meal! Steak and spinach are both excellent sources of 'iron' in our diet.

For 2
2 tbsp extra-virgin olive oil
1 large red onion, peeled and chopped
1 medium garlic clove, peeled and chopped
400 grams minute steak (approximately 4 thin steaks)
4 slices fresh root ginger, peeled and finely chopped
100 grams spinach leaves
2 medium plum vine tomatoes, sliced
1 tbsp sesame seeds
freshly ground black pepper

- Heat the extra-virgin olive oil in a large frying pan and add the onions. Cook for about 5 minutes on low heat.
- Add the garlic, steaks and ginger, and cook over high heat for 3–4 minutes, turning the steaks once.
- Add the spinach and tomato slices, sprinkle over the sesame seeds, and season to taste.
- Heat for a further 2–3 minutes, then serve immediately.

CARBOHYDRATE CONTENT PER SERVING: 8 GRAMS

Beef jalfrezi curry with peppers

Mustard is actually a member of the cabbage family! Originally the seeds were mixed with grape must – hence the name 'mustard'.

For 2
5 tbsp extra-virgin olive oil
250 grams minute steak, thinly sliced
1 tsp black mustard seeds
1 tsp cumin seeds
1 medium red onion, peeled and chopped
1 medium garlic clove, peeled and finely chopped
1 tbsp medium curry powder
2 tsp plain flour
75 ml beef stock
3 slices fresh ginger root, peeled and finely chopped
1 medium red pepper, deseeded and finely sliced
1 medium green pepper, deseeded and finely sliced
1 tbsp chopped fresh coriander
freshly ground black pepper
100 grams wild rocket leaves

- Heat 2 tablespoons extra-virgin olive oil in a large frying pan and stir-fry the steak for 3–4 minutes, then remove from the pan and set aside.

- Wipe the pan dry then stir-fry the mustard and cumin seeds, then remove from the pan and set aside.
- Add the remaining extra-virgin olive oil to the pan and sauté the onion and garlic for 3–4 minutes.
- Remove from the heat, stir in the curry powder and flour, then gradually stir in the stock.
- Return the steak to the pan, stir in the ginger, peppers, coriander, mustard and cumin seeds, and simmer gently for 4–5 minutes.
- Season to taste and serve immediately with wild rocket.

CARBOHYDRATE CONTENT PER SERVING: 12 GRAMS

Quick method

For 2

250 grams minute steak, thinly sliced
2 tbsp extra-virgin olive oil
1 medium garlic clove, peeled and finely chopped
1 medium red pepper, deseeded and finely sliced
1 medium green pepper, deseeded and finely sliced
200 grams Loyd Grossman jalfrezi curry sauce
100 grams wild rocket leaves
freshly ground black pepper

- Heat the extra-virgin olive oil in a wok and stir-fry the sliced steak and garlic for 3–4 minutes.
- Add the peppers and stir-fry for a further minute, then mix in the jalfrezi curry sauce and heat through for 3 minutes.
- Serve immediately with wild rocket and season to taste with freshly ground black pepper.

CARBOHYDRATE CONTENT PER SERVING: 12 GRAMS

Chicken satay with lime

Freshly ground black pepper is included in many recipes, not just for taste, but also because ground black pepper contains a high concentration of the mineral chromium, which we need for the functioning of our pancreas and which is important in the prevention of diabetes.

For 2
250 grams chicken breast fillets, skinned and cubed
200 grams fresh spinach leaves
1 lime quartered
freshly ground black pepper

Marinade
2 shallots, peeled and diced
1 garlic clove, peeled and crushed
2 tsp medium curry powder
2 tbsp peanut butter
1 tbsp liquid honey
3 tbsp soy sauce

- Mix together the ingredients for the marinade and marinate the chicken for 3–4 hours.
- Soak two wooden skewers in cold water for 5–10 minutes before cooking.
- Thread the chicken cubes onto the wooden skewers.
- Grill (or barbecue) under a hot grill (8–10 cm from the grill) for 8–10 minutes, turning regularly.

At the same time
- Lightly steam the spinach for 4–5 minutes or microwave the spinach for 3–4 minutes.

- Serve the chicken satay kebabs on a bed of spinach, drizzle over some freshly squeezed lime juice and season to taste.

CARBOHYDRATE CONTENT PER SERVING: 10 GRAMS

Quick method

For 2
250 grams chicken breast fillets, skinned and cubed
200 grams Loyd Grossman satay sauce
200 grams fresh spinach leaves
1 lime, quartered
freshly ground black pepper

- Soak the wooden skewers in cold water for 5–10 minutes before cooking.
- Mix the chicken cubes with the satay sauce, then thread the cubes onto the wooden skewers.
- Grill (or barbecue) under a hot grill (8–10 cm from the grill) for 8–10 minutes, turning regularly.

At the same time
- Lightly steam the spinach for 4–5 minutes or microwave the spinach for 3–4 minutes.

- Serve the chicken satay kebabs on a bed of spinach, drizzle over some freshly squeezed lime juice, and season to taste.

CARBOHYDRATE CONTENT PER SERVING: 17 GRAMS

Thai chicken with lemongrass and ginger

Ginger has been recognised for its medicinal properties since ancient times. It is said to improve circulation and prevent blood coagulation, as well as improve digestion.

For 2
250 grams chicken breast fillets
50 grams butter, cubed
3 tbsp extra-virgin olive oil
1 medium red onion, peeled and sliced
1 medium garlic clove, peeled and finely sliced
2 stalks lemongrass, husk removed and finely chopped

1 green chilli, deseeded and chopped finely (optional)
3 slices fresh ginger root, peeled and finely chopped
1 tbsp tamarind paste
1 medium red pepper, deseeded and sliced
1 medium green pepper, deseeded and sliced
100 grams mangetout
400 ml coconut milk
freshly ground black pepper

- Place the chicken breast fillets in a shallow baking dish, dot with butter cubes and cover with pierced aluminium foil.
- Cook in the centre of a pre-heated oven at 180°C (gas 4) for 35–40 minutes, then remove from the oven, allow to cool and slice into strips.
- Heat the extra-virgin olive oil in a wok and stir-fry the onion and garlic for 2–3 minutes.
- Add the lemon grass, chilli, ginger and tamarind paste.
- Add the peppers and mangetout and stir-fry for a further 2 minutes.
- Stir in the coconut milk and chicken, and simmer gently for 10 minutes, then serve immediately. Season to taste with freshly ground black pepper.

CARBOHYDRATE CONTENT PER SERVING: 17 GRAMS

Quick method
For 2
250 grams chicken breast fillets
50 grams butter, cubed
1 tbsp extra-virgin olive oil
1 medium red onion, peeled and sliced
1 medium garlic clove, peeled and finely sliced
1 medium red pepper, deseeded and sliced
1 medium green pepper, deseeded and sliced

100 grams mangetout
75 grams Sharwoods Thai lemongrass and ginger sauce
freshly ground black pepper

- Place the chicken breast fillets in a shallow baking dish, dot with butter cubes and cover with pierced aluminium foil.
- Cook in the centre of a pre-heated oven at 180°C (gas 4) for 35–40 minutes, then remove from the oven, allow to cool and slice.

Or
- Use 2 ready-cooked chicken breast fillets from the supermarket, sliced.
- Heat the extra-virgin olive oil in a wok and stir-fry the onion and garlic for 2–3 minutes.
- Add the peppers and mangetout and stir-fry for a further 2 minutes.
- Stir in the sauce and chicken, simmer for 2–3 minutes, then serve immediately.
- Season to taste with freshly ground black pepper.

CARBOHYDRATE CONTENT PER SERVING: 14 GRAMS

Chicken korma with mangetout and broccoli

Broccoli is a particularly rich source of folate and calcium, as well as the antioxidant vitamin C.

For 2
250 grams chicken breast fillets
50 grams butter, cubed
2 tbsp extra-virgin olive oil
1 medium red onion, peeled and diced
1 garlic clove, peeled and finely chopped
2 green cardamom pods
2 slices fresh root ginger, peeled and finely chopped
1 tsp ground cumin

1 tsp dried coriander
1 tsp garam masala
½ tsp chilli powder
150 ml natural yoghurt
100 grams mangetout
100 grams broccoli florets
freshly ground black pepper

- Place the chicken breast fillets in a shallow baking dish, dot with butter cubes and cover with pierced aluminium foil.
- Cook in the centre of a pre-heated oven at 180°C (gas 4) for 35–40 minutes, then remove from the oven, allow to cool and slice.

At the same time
- Heat the extra-virgin olive oil in a wok and sauté the onion and garlic for 2-3 minutes.
- Stir in the cardamom, ginger, cumin, coriander, garam masala and chilli powder.
- Stir in the yoghurt, return the chicken strips to the pan and simmer very gently for 3–4 minutes. Do not boil, as it will ruin the sauce!

At the same time
- Lightly steam the mangetout for 5 minutes and the broccoli for 10 minutes, or microwave the mangetout and broccoli for 3–4 minutes.
- Season to taste and serve immediately.

CARBOHYDRATE CONTENT PER SERVING: 11 GRAMS

Quick method
For 2
250 grams chicken breast fillets
50 grams butter, cubed
1 tbsp extra-virgin olive oil

100 grams mangetout
100 grams broccoli florets
200 grams of Loyd Grossman korma sauce
freshly ground black pepper

- Place the chicken breast fillets in a shallow baking dish, dot with butter cubes and cover with pierced aluminium foil.
- Cook in the centre of a pre-heated oven at 180°C (gas 4) for 35–40 minutes, then remove from the oven, allow to cool and slice.

Or
- Use 2 ready-cooked chicken breast fillets from the supermarket, sliced.
- Heat the extra-virgin olive oil in a wok and stir-fry the mangetout and broccoli for 2–3 minutes.
- Add the korma sauce and cooked chicken, and simmer for 3–4 minutes. Do not boil, as it will ruin the sauce!
- Season to taste with freshly ground black pepper and serve immediately.

CARBOHYDRATE CONTENT PER SERVING: 21 GRAMS

Lamb tikka masala with broccoli

There is no quick way to make tikka masala apart from using a prepared sauce. The method involves initially making a tandoori marinade and marinating the lamb for 24 hours. Then a masala sauce is made (using 14 ingredients, mostly specialised). So if you would like to enjoy a quick-and-easy tikka masala as a mid-week meal, I'm afraid you will have to settle for a prepared sauce.

For 2
2 tbsp extra-virgin olive oil
250 grams lean lamb fillet, sliced

1 slice fresh root ginger, peeled and finely chopped
200 grams Loyd Grossman tikka masala sauce
100 grams broccoli florets
freshly ground black pepper

- Heat the extra-virgin olive oil in a wok and stir-fry the sliced lamb and ginger for 2–3 minutes.
- Stir in the tikka masala sauce and simmer gently for 3–4 minutes.

At the same time
- Lightly steam the broccoli for 10 minutes or microwave the broccoli for 3–4 minutes.
- Season to taste and serve immediately.

CARBOHYDRATE CONTENT PER SERVING: 14 GRAMS

Turkey teriyaki

Turkey breast is available ready-sliced into 'steaks' (approximately 1 cm thick) from most supermarkets. It is very lean, relatively inexpensive, absorbs flavours wonderfully, contains virtually no carbohydrates and cooks quickly.

For 2
2 tbsp mirin (sweet rice wine)
2 tbsp shoyu (Japanese soy sauce)
2 tbsp saki
2 slices fresh ginger root, peeled and finely chopped
300 grams sliced turkey breast (approximately)
50 grams unsalted butter
100 grams spinach leaves
freshly ground black pepper

- Mix together the mirin, shoyu, saki and ginger in a shallow baking dish and marinate the sliced turkey breast for 20 minutes.

- Cover with pierced aluminium foil and cook in the centre of a pre-heated oven at 180°C (gas 4) for 30–35 minutes.

Just before the turkey is cooked
- Melt the butter in a medium frying pan and gently sauté the spinach leaves for 1–2 minutes until they just begin to soften.
- Season to taste and serve the turkey immediately on a bed of sautéed spinach leaves.

CARBOHYDRATE CONTENT PER SERVING: 4 GRAMS

Meatballs with tomato and basil sauce

Tomatoes are a rich source of the important antioxidant lycopene, which clears free radicals and helps to prevent the ageing process.

For 2
250 grams lean minced beef
1 medium red onion, peeled and finely diced
1 garlic clove, peeled and finely chopped
1 egg, beaten
2 tbsp chopped fresh basil leaves
tomato sauce (pages 274–75)
100 grams French beans
100 grams yellow baby squash, halved
freshly ground black pepper
1 tbsp chopped chives (optional)

- Mix together the mince, onion, garlic, egg, and 1 tablespoon of chopped fresh basil in a medium mixing bowl.
- Form the mixture into small balls, 3–4 cm in diameter.
- Place on a baking tray, and cook under a hot grill

199

(approx 8–10 cm from the grill) for about 8 minutes, turning 2–3 times.

At the same time
- Make the tomato sauce, and
- Lightly steam the French beans and yellow squash for 10 minutes or microwave the vegetables for 3–4 minutes.
- Serve the meatballs, spoon over some tomato sauce, and add the vegetables.
- Season to taste and garnish with chopped chives

CARBOHYDRATE CONTENT PER SERVING: 12 GRAMS
(ONLY 6 GRAMS WITHOUT TOMATO SAUCE)

Gammon steaks with honey

With essential amino acids and vitamin B_1 from gammon and vitamin C from French beans and lemon juice, this is a very nutritious meal.

For 2
2 gammon steaks, approximately 150 grams each
2 tbsp extra-virgin olive oil
75 grams French beans
50 grams unsalted butter
2 tbsp freshly squeezed lemon juice
freshly ground black pepper

Marinade
1 tbsp liquid honey
2 tbsp freshly squeezed orange juice
1 tbsp sesame seeds
1 garlic clove, peeled and finely chopped
3 slices fresh root ginger, peeled and finely chopped

- Mix together the honey, orange juice, sesame seeds, garlic and ginger in a wide shallow dish.

- Place the gammon steaks in the marinade and marinate for at least 20 minutes. (The perfect solution is to prepare the marinade the previous evening and marinate the gammon overnight.)
- Heat the extra-virgin olive oil in a large frying pan and fry the gammon steaks for 5–6 minutes, turning once.

At the same time
- Microwave the French beans for 3–4 minutes on 'high' and allow to stand for 1 minute or lightly steam the French beans for 8–10 minutes.

And
- Prepare the lemon butter sauce (page 263).

- Season to taste with freshly ground black pepper, then serve the honey gammon steaks with the French beans, drizzling the lemon butter sauce over the beans.

CARBOHYDRATE CONTENT PER SERVING: 9 GRAMS

Prawn omelette

Parsley is a rich source of vitamins A and C, which are important antioxidants in our diet.

For 2
2 tbsp extra-virgin olive oil
1 shallot, peeled and finely chopped
50 grams cooked and peeled prawns
1 tbsp single cream
1 tbsp fresh parsley, finely chopped
15 grams butter
4 large free-range eggs, beaten
freshly ground black pepper
fresh dill sprigs, to garnish

- Heat the virgin olive oil in a small saucepan and sauté the shallot for 1 minute.
- Lower the heat, add the prawns, and cook for 1–2 minutes, then stir in the cream and parsley and gently heat through for a further minute.

At the same time
- Heat the butter in a (preferably) non-stick medium frying pan, pour in the egg mixture, and cook until the omelette is almost cooked through, but is still creamy on the surface.
- Spoon the prawn mixture onto one half of the omelette, fold in half, and serve immediately.
- Season to taste and garnish with sprigs of fresh dill.

CARBOHYDRATE CONTENT PER SERVING: 2 GRAMS

Turkey in cherry tomato and chilli sauce

Chillies are actually members of the pepper (or capsicum) family and provide a rich source of vitamins A and C as well as the mineral iron.

For 2
2 tbsp extra-virgin olive oil
250 grams turkey breast fillets, sliced into thin strips
2 tbsp tomato purée
10 cherry tomatoes, halved
1 large red chilli, deseeded and finely chopped
50 ml chicken stock
1 tbsp chopped fresh oregano (or 2 tsp dried oregano)
100 grams wild rocket

- Heat the extra-virgin olive oil in a wok, then stir-fry the sliced turkey for 3–4 minutes.
- Stir in the tomato purée, cherry tomatoes, chilli and chicken stock.

- Add the fresh (or dried) oregano.
- Simmer gently for 7–8 minutes, then serve on a bed of wild rocket.

CARBOHYDRATE CONTENT PER SERVING: 9 GRAMS

Quick method
For 2

2 tbsp extra-virgin olive oil
250 grams turkey breast fillets, sliced into thin strips
200 grams of SACLA whole cherry tomatoes and red chilli sauce
1 tbsp chopped fresh oregano (or 2 tsp dried oregano)
100 grams wild rocket

- Heat the virgin olive oil in a wok, then stir-fry the sliced turkey for 3–4 minutes.
- Stir in the tomato and chilli sauce and add the fresh oregano.
- Simmer gently for 3–4 minutes, then serve on a bed of wild rocket.

CARBOHYDRATE CONTENT PER SERVING: 7 GRAMS

Thai koftas with mango raita

This can be enjoyed equally successfully with a commercial raita to save time but remember to check the carbohydrate content.

For 2

1½ tbsp Schwartz Thai crushed spices
250 grams lean beef minced steak
1 large free-range egg, beaten
1 medium red onion, peeled and finely diced
1 large garlic clove, peeled and grated
freshly ground black pepper

crispy herb salad (page 263)
mango raita (page 275)

- Soak two wooden skewers in water for at least 20 minutes before use.
- Dry stir-fry the Thai crushed spices in a small frying pan for about a minute.
- Mix together the spices, beef mince, ½ beaten egg, onion and garlic in a medium bowl.
- Form the beef mixture into 'sausage shapes' around the kebab skewers, cover and cool in the fridge for at least 10 minutes.
- Place a well-oiled sheet of baking paper on the grill tray and lay the kebabs on the tray in a single layer.
- Grill on high for 10–12 minutes, no closer than 8–10 cm from the grill, turning the kebabs frequently.

At the same time
- Prepare the mango raita.
- Season the kebabs to taste and serve immediately with mango raita and crispy herb salad.

CARBOHYDRATE CONTENT PER SERVING: 16 GRAMS

Turkey bolognaise with peppers

Peppers provide a rich source of vitamins A and C, especially red peppers.

For 2
4 tbsp extra-virgin olive oil
250 grams turkey breast fillets, sliced into thin strips
1 medium red onion, peeled and chopped
1 garlic clove, peeled and chopped
2 tbsp tomato purée
100 ml chicken stock
1 small red pepper, deseeded and sliced

1 small yellow pepper, deseeded and sliced
3 medium courgettes, sliced thickly on the diagonal
2 slices fresh ginger, peeled and chopped
100 grams baby spinach leaves, washed

- Heat 2 tablespoons of extra-virgin olive oil in a large frying pan and stir-fry the sliced turkey for 3–4 minutes, then remove from the pan, set aside and cover.
- Heat the remaining extra-virgin olive oil in the pan and sauté the onion and garlic for 2–3 minutes.
- Remove from the heat and stir in the tomato purée and stock.
- Return to the heat and simmer the peppers, courgettes and ginger for 3–4 minutes.
- Return the sliced turkey to the pan and simmer gently for 3–4 minutes, season to taste, and serve on a bed of baby spinach leaves.

CARBOHYDRATE CONTENT PER SERVING: 14 GRAMS

Quick method

For 2

2 tablespoons extra-virgin olive oil
250 grams turkey breast fillets, sliced into thin strips
320-gram jar Dolmio bolognaise sauce
50 ml water
1 small red pepper, deseeded and sliced
1 small yellow pepper, deseeded and sliced
3 medium courgettes, sliced thickly on the diagonal
2 slices fresh ginger, peeled and chopped
100 grams baby spinach leaves

- Heat the extra-virgin olive oil in a large frying pan and stir-fry the sliced turkey for 3–4 minutes.
- Stir in the bolognaise sauce and water, then add the peppers, courgettes and ginger.

- Simmer gently for 7–8 minutes, season to taste, and serve on a bed of baby spinach leaves.

CARBOHYDRATE CONTENT PER SERVING: 16 GRAMS

Sesame beef with ginger and lemon grass

Sesame seeds provide the essential omega-6 fatty acids in our diet.

For 2
4 tbsp extra-virgin olive oil
250 grams minute steak, sliced into strips
4 slices fresh root ginger, peeled and chopped
2 stalks lemongrass, dehusked and finely chopped
1 tbsp sesame seeds
75 grams carrot, peeled and sliced julienne
75 grams mangetout
1 small red chilli, deseeded and finely chopped
1 medium red pepper, deseeded and finely sliced
1 tbsp chopped fresh chives, to garnish

- Heat 2 tablespoons of the extra-virgin olive oil in a medium frying pan and gently stir-fry the minute steak for 2–3 minutes.
- Add the ginger, lemon grass and sesame seeds and stir-fry for a further 3-4 minutes.

At the same time
- Heat the remaining 2 tablespoons of virgin olive oil in a wok and stir-fry the carrot, mangetout, chilli and pepper for 3–4 minutes.

- Serve the sesame beef with the vegetables, garnished with chopped chives.

CARBOHYDRATE CONTENT PER SERVING: 9 GRAMS

Quick method

For 2

2 tbsp extra-virgin olive oil
250 grams minute steak, sliced into strips
4 slices fresh root ginger, peeled and chopped
1 tbsp sesame seeds
2 tbsp Sharwoods sweet chilli and lemon grass sauce
300-gram packet of mixed stir-fry vegetables
1 tbsp chopped fresh chives, to garnish

- Heat 2 tablespoons of the extra-virgin olive oil in a medium frying pan, and gently fry the minute steak, ginger and sesame seeds for 3–4 minutes.
- Add the ginger and lemon grass sauce and gently simmer for a further 3–4 minutes.

At the same time
- Heat the remaining 2 tablespoons of virgin olive oil in a wok and stir-fry the vegetables for 2–3 minutes.
- Serve the sesame beef with the vegetables, garnished with chopped chives.

CARBOHYDRATE CONTENT PER SERVING: 14 GRAMS

Spicy scrambled eggs

This delicious meal is nutritionally complete with essential amino acids and vitamin B_{12} from eggs, vitamin B and potassium from onions, and vitamins A and C from tomatoes and chilli.

For 2

2 tbsp extra-virgin olive oil
1 small onion (or 2 shallots), peeled and finely chopped
½ small red chilli, deseeded and finely chopped (optional)
1 small plum tomato, deseeded and chopped finely
2 tsp chopped fresh coriander leaves

¼ tsp ground cumin
½ tsp ground ginger
pinch ground turmeric
4 large free-range eggs, beaten
freshly ground black pepper

- Heat the virgin olive oil in a medium frying pan and sauté the onion (or shallots).
- Add the chilli, tomato, coriander and spices and stir-fry for 2-3 minutes.
- Stir in the eggs, and cook gently over a low heat, stirring regularly.
- Season to taste and serve immediately.

CARBOHYDRATE CONTENT PER SERVING: 4 GRAMS

Sweet and sour beef with mangetout

'Forbidden' foods like sugar can, of course, be included in your diet – in small quantities. Fifteen grams of carbohydrates in a tablespoon of sugar divided between two (or four) people will not significantly affect your diet (as compared to 60 grams of sugar in a single bar of chocolate!).

For 2
4 tbsp extra-virgin olive oil
250 grams minute steak
1 medium red onion, peeled and chopped
1 garlic clove, peeled and finely chopped
1 medium red pepper, deseeded and thinly sliced
75 grams mangetout
2 slices root ginger, peeled and finely chopped
freshly ground black pepper

Sweet and sour sauce

1 tbsp granulated sugar
1 tbsp white wine vinegar

50 ml beef stock
1 tsp tomato purée
2 tsp cornflour

- To make the sauce mix together the sugar, wine
  vinegar, stock and tomato purée in a medium bowl
  and gradually stir in the cornflour to form an even
  paste.
- Heat 2 tablespoons extra-virgin olive oil in a
  medium frying pan and stir-fry the steak for 3–4
  minutes, turning once.
- Remove the steak from the pan, slice thinly and set
  aside.
- Heat the remaining olive oil in the pan and sauté
  the onion and garlic for 1-2 minutes.
- Add the pepper, mangetout and ginger, and stir-fry
  for a further 2–3 minutes.
- Return the steak to the pan, stir in the sweet and
  sour sauce, and simmer gently for 2–3 minutes.
- Season to taste and serve immediately.

CARBOHYDRATE CONTENT PER SERVING: 19 GRAMS

Quick method

For 2

4 tbsp extra-virgin olive oil
250 grams minute steak
1 medium red onion, peeled and chopped
1 garlic clove, peeled and finely chopped
1 medium red pepper, deseeded and thinly sliced
75 grams mangetout
2 slices ginger root, peeled and finely chopped
80 grams (½ jar) of Sharwood's sweet and sour sauce
freshly ground black pepper

- Heat 2 tablespoons olive oil in a medium frying pan
  and stir-fry the steak for 3–4 minutes, turning once.

- Remove the steak from the pan, slice thinly and set aside.
- Heat the remaining olive oil in the pan and sauté the onion and garlic for 1–2 minutes.
- Add the pepper, mangetout and ginger, and stir-fry for a further 2–3 minutes.
- Return the steak to the pan, stir in the sweet and sour sauce and simmer for 2–3 minutes.
- Season to taste and serve immediately.

CARBOHYDRATE CONTENT PER SERVING: 18 GRAMS

Gammon and aubergine with herbs

Aubergines are a rich source of the antioxidant vitamin E.

For 2
5 tbsp extra-virgin olive oil
2 gammon steaks (approx 125 grams each)
1 medium aubergine (approx 250 grams), sliced lengthways into 1-cm slices
1 tbsp chopped fresh coriander
1 tbsp chopped fresh basil
150 grams grated cheese of choice (Edam, Gouda or Emmental are delicious in this recipe)
freshly ground black pepper
1 tbsp chopped fresh chives

- Heat 2 tablespoons of extra-virgin olive oil in a large frying pan and fry the gammon steaks.

At the same time
- Place the aubergine slices in a single layer on a baking tray, drizzle with the remaining extra-virgin olive oil, and cook under a hot grill, no closer than 8 cm from the grill, for 2 minutes, then turn over, drizzle with more olive oil, and grill for a further 2 minutes.

- Top the aubergine slices with herbs and cheese and grill for a final 2 minutes.
- Serve immediately with the gammon, season to taste and garnish with chopped chives.

CARBOHYDRATE CONTENT PER SERVING: 4 GRAMS

Salmon with Bocconcini and basil

Salmon is a marvellous source of so many essential nutrients, including amino acids, essential omega-3 fatty acids, vitamin D, vitamin E and calcium.

For 2
2 salmon fillets, about 150 grams each
25 grams unsalted butter, cubed
1 tbsp chopped fresh basil (optional)
4–6 thin slices Bocconcini cheese
100 grams mangetout
freshly ground black pepper

- Place the salmon fillets in a shallow, oven-safe dish, dot with butter cubes, cover with pierced aluminium foil and cook in the centre of a pre-heated oven at 180°C (gas 4) for about 12 minutes.
- Remove from the oven, top the fillets with chopped fresh basil and 2–3 slices of Bocconcini cheese and return to the oven for 3–4 minutes.

At the same time
- Place the mangetout in a microwave-safe container, add 1 tablespoon of water, cover and cook on high for 2½ minutes (depending on the power of the oven) or lightly steam the mangetout for 5 minutes.
- Serve the salmon with the mangetout and season to taste with freshly ground black pepper.

CARBOHYDRATE CONTENT PER SERVING: 2 GRAMS

211

Peking duck

Duck and orange complement one another nutritionally as well as gastronomically: duck provides all essential amino acids and orange provides the missing vitamin C.

For 2

2 tbsp dry sherry
1 tbsp liquid honey
1 tbsp light soy sauce
3 tbsp freshly squeezed orange juice (or packaged orange juice if necessary)
2 slices fresh ginger root, peeled and finely chopped
2 duck breasts (approximately 150 grams each)
baby leeks in lemon butter sauce (pages 262–63)
freshly ground black pepper
2 spring onions, finely sliced lengthways, to garnish

- Mix together the sherry, honey, soy sauce, orange juice and ginger, and marinate the duck breasts for as long as possible (at least 20 minutes). If you can plan ahead and marinate the duck breasts overnight in the fridge that would be ideal.
- Place the duck breasts on a rack in a roasting tin, pour over the remaining marinade and roast in the centre of a pre-heated oven at 180°C (gas 4) for 30–35 minutes.
- Remove the duck from the oven, allow to cool for 10–15 minutes then carve into thin slices.

At the same time
- Prepare the baby leeks in lemon butter sauce.

- Serve the duck breast slices on a bed of leeks, season to taste and garnish with chopped spring onions.

CARBOHYDRATE CONTENT PER SERVING: 10 GRAMS

Plaice with olives

The healthy properties of olives have been recognised for centuries. They are a rich source of antioxidant polyphenols, vitamin E and the mineral magnesium.

For 2
2 tbsp extra-virgin olive oil
3 shallots, peeled and diced
1 garlic clove, peeled and finely chopped
1 tbsp tomato purée
1 tbsp dry sherry
1 tsp Worcestershire sauce
8–10 green olives
100 ml fish stock
2 plaice fillets
75 grams broccoli florets
75 grams yellow squash, halved lengthways
freshly ground black pepper

- Heat the extra-virgin olive oil in a medium frying pan and sauté the shallots and garlic for 1–2 minutes.
- Stir in the tomato purée, sherry, Worcestershire sauce, olives and stock, then add the plaice fillets to the sauce.
- Cover and simmer gently for 10–12 minutes.

At the same time
- Lightly steam the broccoli and yellow squash for 3–4 minutes or microwave for 3–4 minutes.

- Season to taste and serve immediately.

Quicker method
It is almost impossible to prepare this meal even faster, but this is a slightly quicker method.

- Prepare the sauce as above but instead of poaching

the plaice fillets in the sauce, lay the fillets in a shallow, microwave-safe dish, cover and cook on high for 2 minutes.

- Allow to stand for 1 minute (no longer or the fish will overcook) and serve immediately.
- Pour the sauce over the fillets and season to taste.

CARBOHYDRATE CONTENT PER SERVING: 6 GRAMS

Balti chicken

Cooking does not have to follow strict rules. This recipe combines Indian spices with chicken and oyster sauce with vegetables. It can be cooked in less than 15 minutes and tastes delicious.

For 2
2 tbsp Schwartz balti crushed curry spices
4 tbsp extra-virgin olive oil
150–200 grams chicken breast, sliced into thin strips
2 spring onions, chopped into 3–4cm lengths on the diagonal
2 garlic cloves, peeled and finely chopped
3 large courgettes, chopped lengthways
1 medium green pepper, deseeded and sliced into thin strips
3 slices root ginger, peeled and finely chopped
1 tbsp oyster sauce
50 ml water
freshly ground black pepper

- Dry stir-fry the spices for 1 minute in a wok, then remove from the wok and set aside.
- Heat 2 tablespoons of extra-virgin olive oil in the wok and stir-fry the chicken for 3–4 minutes.
- Stir in the spices, and stir-fry for a further 1–2 minutes.

At the same time
- Heat the remaining 2 tablespoons of extra-virgin olive oil in a separate frying pan and stir-fry the spring onions, garlic, courgettes, pepper and ginger for 3–4 minutes.
- Stir in the oyster sauce and water and heat gently for a further minute.
- Serve the vegetables with the chicken and season to taste.

CARBOHYDRATE CONTENT PER SERVING: 6 GRAMS

Balti pork

For 2
As for balti chicken (pages 214–15), substituting the chicken with 3 medium boneless pork chops, sliced into strips.

CARBOHYDRATE CONTENT PER SERVING: 6 GRAMS

Balti beef

For 2
As for balti chicken (pages 214–15), substituting the chicken with 150-200 grams of minute steak, sliced into strips.

CARBOHYDRATE CONTENT PER SERVING: 6 GRAMS

Grilled ham with mozzarella, basil and cherry tomatoes

Think laterally! You don't really need bread, it just provides the base for other foods; arrange the food in a different way, and the bread is completely unnecessary. In this simple recipe, the thick ham provides the base of the dish, and the meal tastes much better than the comparable 'toastie'.

For 2
2 large thick slices shoulder ham
6 cherry tomatoes, sliced
1 tbsp chopped fresh basil
100 grams mozzarella cheese, sliced
1 tbsp balsamic vinegar
freshly ground black pepper

- Cover a grill tray with aluminium foil and drizzle over a little extra-virgin olive oil.
- Place the thick slices of ham separately on the foil.
- Top the ham with cherry tomatoes, basil and mozzarella cheese, and grill (no closer than 8–10 cm from the heat) until the cheese 'bubbles'.
- Transfer the ham to warm plates, drizzle over the balsamic vinegar and season to taste.

CARBOHYDRATE CONTENT PER SERVING: 3 GRAMS

Swedish meatballs with herbs

This recipe can be made with purely beef, pork, lamb or turkey mince, but the combination of beef with pork is a delicious alternative.

For 2
150 grams lean minced pork
100 grams lean minced beef
1 large, free-range egg, beaten
½ tbsp chopped fresh basil (or ½ tsp dried basil)
½ tbsp chopped fresh coriander (or ½ tsp dried coriander)
2 tsp Worcestershire sauce
1 garlic clove, peeled and crushed
1 spring onion, sliced lengthways into thin strips
2 slices fresh root ginger, peeled and sliced julienne, to garnish
crispy herb salad (page 263)

- Mix together the mince, egg, herbs, Worcestershire sauce and garlic in a medium mixing bowl.
- Form the mixture into small balls 3–4 cm in diameter. Be careful not to make the meatballs too large or it will seriously increase the time required for cooking.
- Grill under a hot grill (no closer then 8–10 cm from the grill) for about 10 minutes, turning frequently.
- Serve immediately with a crispy herb salad, garnished with spring onion and ginger.

Quicker method

Meatballs are available commercially and although they tend to contain some carbohydrates, this is usually no more than 6 grams per 100 grams so it will not ruin the diet. As the crispy herb salad can also be purchased ready-made, this delicious meal can be on the table within about 10 minutes.

CARBOHYDRATE CONTENT PER SERVING: 7 GRAMS (HOME-MADE)
16 GRAMS (WITH COMMERCIAL MEATBALLS)

Eggs Benedict

This recipe is not 'fast' enough to be practical on a normal busy weekday unless you have the time to prepare the Hollandaise sauce on the previous evening; however it is a delicious start to the weekend when a little more time is available to make the Hollandaise sauce. The classic recipe includes Canadian bacon, however this version incorporates proscuitto for a lighter flavour, but obviously unsmoked bacon is an acceptable alternative.

For 2
Hollandaise sauce
1 English muffin
50 grams proscuitto
2 large free-range eggs, poached
chopped fresh chives, to garnish

- Halve the muffin and toast each half lightly. Lay the proscuitto on each half muffin.

At the same time
- Poach the eggs (pages 89–90).
- Place the drained poached eggs on the ham, and top with Hollandaise sauce, garnished with chopped chives.

Quicker method

If you don't have time to make a home-made Hollandaise sauce, use a commercial variety. Not quite as good as home-made, but there are many very acceptable brands of Hollandaise sauce available and you will still enjoy a tasty and highly nutritious meal to complement your diet. But be careful! Commercial Hollandaise sauce usually contains about 8 grams of carbohydrates per 100 grams; however some brands have a much higher carbohydrate content. Read the label to check!

CARBOHYDRATE CONTENT PER SERVING: WITH HOME-MADE HOLLANDAISE SAUCE 15 GRAMS (INCLUDING MUFFIN); WITH COMMERCIAL HOLLANDAISE SAUCE 23 GRAMS (INCLUDING MUFFIN)

Really fast suppers

Really fast suppers are those ready in less than 15 minutes. Obviously the meal has to be simple but that doesn't mean we have to compromise on taste or nutrition. It is very easy to enjoy delicious meals in less than 15 minutes *providing you have the correct ingredients,* and if you want to keep healthy you have to maintain a supply of fresh vegetables. They can be purchased ready-prepared from the supermarket which removes the preparation time so we are left with only cooking time. To retain most of their essential healthy nutrients, vegetables should be either steamed, stir-fried or cooked by microwave. Fortunately these also happen to be the quickest methods of cooking vegetables.

Obviously, with this significant time constraint, the meals have to be simple with relatively few ingredients which should be selected on the basis of taste and nutrition.

Peppered smoked ham with spinach and ricotta

Spinach provides iron and folate, both of which are essential for the formation of blood cells in the body, as well as antioxidant vitamins C and E.

For 2
½ tbsp sesame seeds (optional)
2 tbsp extra-virgin olive oil
75 grams baby spinach leaves
1 garlic clove, peeled and finely chopped
50 grams ricotta cheese, 'crumbled'
4 thick slices pre-cooked peppered, smoked ham
freshly ground black pepper

- Dry stir-fry the sesame seeds in a medium frying pan (or wok) for 1 minute.
- Heat the extra-virgin olive oil in the pan (or wok) and stir-fry the spinach and garlic for about 1 minute.
- Stir in the ricotta cheese and cook for a further minute.
- Season to taste with freshly ground black pepper and serve immediately with pre-cooked peppered smoked ham.

CARBOHYDRATE CONTENT PER SERVING: 2 GRAMS

Steak with cherry tomatoes, basil and coriander

This meal provides vitamin A from tomatoes and even more antioxidants from basil and coriander.

For 2
2 tbsp extra-virgin olive oil
250 grams minute steak
cherry tomatoes with basil and coriander (page 262)
freshly ground black pepper

• Heat the extra-virgin olive oil in a large frying pan and fry the minute steak for 3–4 minutes, turning once.

At the same time
• Cook the cherry tomatoes with basil and coriander.

• Season to taste and serve immediately.

CARBOHYDRATE CONTENT PER SERVING: 4 GRAMS

Mozzarella and tomato omelette

If possible, try to obtain 'genuine' mozzarella cheese made from buffalo milk.

For 2
4 large free-range eggs, beaten
30 ml full-cream milk
2 tbsp extra-virgin olive oil
1 large plum tomato, thinly sliced
1 tbsp chopped fresh flat-leaf parsley (optional)
100 grams ready-grated mozzarella cheese
freshly ground black pepper
50 grams wild rocket leaves

- Mix together the milk and beaten eggs in a medium bowl.
- Heat the extra-virgin olive oil in a medium frying pan, pour in the egg mixture and cook until the omelette is almost cooked through, but is still creamy on the surface.
- Lay the tomato slices in a single layer on the omelette, sprinkle over the parsley and top with grated mozzarella cheese.
- Place the frying pan under a pre-heated grill (no closer than 8–10 cm from the grill) and grill until the cheese just begins to brown.
- Season to taste and serve immediately with wild rocket.

CARBOHYDRATE CONTENT PER SERVING: 4 GRAMS

Salmon with wild rocket and mint sauce

Mangetout and rocket are both rich sources of vitamin C.

For 2
2 fresh salmon fillets (approximately 150 grams each)
75 grams mangetout
wild rocket and mint sauce (page 276)
freshly ground black pepper

- Place the salmon fillets (or steaks) in a suitable microwave container, cover and cook on high for 2½ minutes. Allow to stand for 1 minute (no longer or they will overcook!).

Or
- Place the salmon fillets on a grill tray and grill under a medium grill (no closer than 8–10 cm from the grill) for 6–8 minutes, turning once.

221

At the same time
- Place the mangetout in a microwave-safe container, add a tbsp water and cook on 'high' for 2½ minutes.

Or
- Lightly steam the mangetout for 4–5 minutes.
- Prepare the wild rocket and mint sauce.
- Serve the salmon with the mangetout, season to taste and top with wild rocket and mint sauce.

CARBOHYDRATE CONTENT PER SERVING: 4 GRAMS

Pork chops with Brussels sprouts and citrus butter sauce

If you don't have time to prepare fresh orange and lemon juice, bottled pure juices are an acceptable alternative.

For 2
2 tbsp extra-virgin olive oil
2 large pork chops (approximately 150 grams each)
Brussels sprouts with orange and lemon butter sauce (pages 260–61)
1 tbsp chopped fresh flat-leaf parsley (optional)
freshly ground black pepper

- Heat the extra-virgin olive oil in a medium frying pan and fry the pork chops for 4–5 minutes, turning once.

Or
- Brush the pork chops with extra-virgin olive oil and grill (no closer than 8–10 cm from the grill) under a hot grill for 4–5 minutes, turning once.

At the same time
- Prepare the Brussels sprouts with orange and lemon butter sauce.

- Serve immediately with the pork chops, sprinkle over the parsley and season to taste with freshly ground black pepper.

CARBOHYDRATE CONTENT PER SERVING: 4 GRAMS

Peppered smoked mackerel with spinach in butter sauce

Never overcook spinach, which destroys the vitamin C and prevents the iron and calcium being effectively absorbed.

For 2
2 medium peppered smoked mackerel fillets, flaked
4 cherry vine tomatoes, halved
2 spring onions, finely chopped
spinach with butter sauce (page 259)

- Mix together the ready-cooked, flaked smoked mackerel with the cherry tomatoes and chopped spring onions in a medium bowl.
- Prepare the spinach with butter sauce.
- Lay a bed of spinach with butter sauce in the centre of each plate and top with the smoked mackerel mixture.

CARBOHYDRATE CONTENT PER SERVING: 3 GRAMS

Bombay turkey breast with watercress and rocket salad

If you prefer the meal less spicy simply halve (or omit) the spices.

For 2

250 grams pre-sliced turkey breast
2 tbsp Schwartz Bombay crushed curry spices
2 tbsp extra-virgin olive oil
100 grams watercress and rocket salad (ready prepared)
1 tbsp mayonnaise

- Slice the turkey breast into thin strips.
- Dry stir-fry the spices for 1 minute in a wok, then remove from the wok and set aside.
- Heat 2 tablespoons of extra-virgin olive oil in the wok and stir-fry the turkey strips for 3-4 minutes.
- Stir in the spices, and stir fry for a further 1-2 minutes.
- Lay a bed of watercress and rocket salad on each plate and top with the Bombay turkey and mayonnaise.

CARBOHYDRATE CONTENT PER SERVING: 3 GRAMS

Chilli prawns

Preparation time of 2–3 minutes. Nutritional value unbeatable!

For 2

100 grams cooked and peeled prawns
1 large plum tomato, diced
2 spring onions, finely chopped
1 tbsp mayonnaise
2 tsp Sharwood's hot chilli sauce
100 grams watercress
freshly ground black pepper

- Rinse the prawns in cold water to remove the overpowering 'salty' taste of the brine in which cooked prawns are usually sold.
- Drain, and pat dry with absorbent paper.

- Mix together the prawns, tomato, spring onions, mayonnaise and chilli sauce in a medium bowl.
- Serve on a bed of watercress and season to taste.

CARBOHYDRATE CONTENT PER SERVING: 3 GRAMS

Chargrilled basil pesto salmon with asparagus

Pine nuts (in basil pesto sauce) are an excellent source of vitamin B_1 and vitamin E.

For 2
1 tbsp extra-virgin olive oil
2 medium salmon fillets or steaks (approximately 150 grams each)
2 tbsp basil pesto sauce, either commercial or home-made (page 275)
8 asparagus spears
50 grams unsalted butter
2 tbsp freshly squeezed lemon juice
freshly ground black pepper

- Brush the salmon fillets (or steaks) with a little extra-virgin olive oil then grill under a hot grill (no closer than 8–10 cm from the grill).
- Coat one side of the salmon with the basil pesto sauce then char-grill for another 2 minutes.

At the same time
- Place the asparagus in the base of a suitable microwave-safe container, arranged with the thick stalks to the outside of the dish and the thin tops facing inwards.
- Add 2 tablespoons water, cover and cook on 'high' for 2–3 minutes, than allow to stand for 1 minute.

Or
- Lightly steam the asparagus for 10–12 minutes.

And
- Heat the butter in a small saucepan, then stir in the lemon juice.

- Serve the salmon with the asparagus and drizzle the lemon butter sauce over the asparagus.

CARBOHYDRATE CONTENT PER SERVING: 4 GRAMS

Ready-prepared meals

Microwavable meals from supermarkets

It is important to consider food in a totally different way if you intend to be healthy on a 'fast food' diet. With a little planning ahead, you will soon realise that health and 'fast food' can easily be combined – providing it is *real* fast food. Microwavable food from supermarkets is the obvious solution. Not the usual polystyrene low-fat, low-taste variety, but rather the delicious meals that are found in other gourmet (and non-diet) sections of the store *and which are actually low in carbohydrate content.* Remember, *diet foods* in the terminology of supermarkets generally means *low-fat* or *low-calorie* foods, which are almost always high-carb foods! And supermarket diet foods always seem to have the same bland taste. Gourmet foods, on the other hand, are exactly the opposite: they are delicious and low in carbohydrates. You will find a good selection of low-carb foods where you least expect on supermarket shelves. For example, who would expect to find delicious low-carb meals in the Indian food section, but there they are – providing you know how to look and *what to look for.*

As a general rule, *avoid the 'diet', low-fat, low-calorie*

section of supermarket microwavable meals because these are almost always high in carbohydrates. Go directly to the gourmet section (including Indian and Chinese cuisine) where you will find the most delicious meals which are also those with least carbohydrates, providing you choose carefully and read the nutrition labels.

Of course you have to know what you are looking for because seemingly comparable meals can have immensely different carbohydrate contents. For example, two very similar supermarket chicken curries may have very different carbohydrate content: Chicken Sag (a blend of spinach, tomatoes and onions, with cumin seeds and green cardamoms) contains less than 15 grams of carbohydrate per 350 gram meal (or less than the amount of carbohydrate in a single slice of bread, to place this in perspective), compared to 79 grams of carbohydrate in an ostensibly similar serving of Chicken Biryani. Indian meals from supermarkets are described in detail on pages 235–37.

Other meals within this category can obviously be divided into those that can be included in a low-carb diet and those that cannot be included. Once again, it must be emphasised that different outlets produce different nutritional combinations of products with similar names; for example, chicken casserole will almost certainly have different carbohydrate and protein content from different outlets. Supermarkets are constantly altering the range of microwavable foods they offer, so you may not find all of the foods in the list available at all outlets. The importance of this list is not to be all-inclusive but merely to demonstrate the types of meals available at any given time and to encourage you, once again, to read the nutritional information on the food label. By this simple method, you will soon differentiate those foods which can be included or excluded from your diet.

Meals which can be included in a low-carb diet

Meal	Weight (g)	Carbs (g)	Protein (g)
Cauliflower cheese	300	12	13
2 chicken breasts with asparagus in Chardonney sauce			
for 2:	560	12	80
per serving:	280	6	40
Paprika beef			
for 2:	550	16	82
per serving:	275	8	41
Butter chicken			
for 2:	350	20	42
per serving:	175	10	21
Braised steak in rich ale sauce with baby onions			
for 2:	440	26	57
per serving:	220	13	29
Chicken breast in creamy white wine and mushroom sauce			
for 2:	450	5	63
per serving:	225	3	32
Barbecue chicken wings	500	20	44
Shepherd's pie	200	21	11
Ready-to-roast chicken breast with cherry tomatoes and mozzarella cheese			

Meal	Weight (g)	Carbs (g)	Protein (g)
for 2:	510	15	97
per serving:	255	8	48
Steak in creamy green peppercorn sauce			
for 2:	400	12	56
per serving:	200	6	28
Salmon in creamy sauce	200	10	12
Chicken casserole	200	22	14
Roast lamb in mint gravy	200	14	14
Liver and onions	200	22	16
Chicken breast escalopes with smoked ham, Cheddar cheese and mushrooms			
for 2:	310	< 1	59
per serving:	155	< 1	30
Barbecue rack of ribs			
for 2:	360	42	43
per serving:	280	21	22
Crispy lemon chicken			
for 2:	300	45	36
per serving:	150	23	18
Minced beef hotpot	200	22	14
Italian fish bake			
for 2:	400	16	48
per serving:	200	8	24
Beef casserole	200	18	14

Meal	Weight (g)	Carbs (g)	Protein (g)
Roast duck à l'orange			
for 2:	540	32	71
per serving:	270	16	36
Braised beef and carrots	200	8	16
Salmon in watercress sauce			
for 2:	400	12	56
per serving:	200	6	28
Haddock fillets in cheese mornay sauce			
for 2:	400	8	56
per serving:	200	4	28
Scottish trout in lemon sauce			
for 2:	400	8	48
per serving:	200	4	24
Salmon in creamy herb sauce with asparagus			
for 2:	370	< 1	46
per serving:	185	< 1	23
Salmon with mustard and dill sauce			
for 2:	380	15	53
per serving:	190	8	27
Chargrilled chicken with peppers, onion and cheese in tomato and basil sauce			
for 2:	470	9	61
per serving:	235	5	30

Meal	Weight (g)	Carbs (g)	Protein (g)
Cottage pie			
for 2:	400	35	22
per serving:	200	18	11
Lamb hotpot			
for 2:	340	44	17
per serving:	170	22	9
Mushroom Stroganoff			
for 2:	400	45	11
per serving:	200	23	6
Haddock pie			
for 2:	400	38	20
per serving:	200	19	10
Ready-to-roast turkey breast			
for 5:	1250	25	238
per serving:	250	5	48
Sausage hotpot			
for 2:	340	48	17
per serving:	170	24	9
Tandoori chicken with spiced couscous			
for 2:	355	36	18
per serving:	178	18	9
Thai-style prawns with cucumber, spring onion and noodles			
for 2:	300	33	12
per serving:	150	17	6

Vegetables to accompany main meals which can be included in a low-carb diet

Meal	Weight (g)	Carbs (g)	Protein (g)
Roasted Mediterranean vegetables			
for 2:	300	20	4
per serving:	150	10	2
Carrot and swede potato mash			
for 2:	450	36	9
per serving:	225	18	5
Cabbage medley (Savoy, spring green and primo cabbage) in cream and onion sauce			
for 2:	300	9	6
per serving:	150	5	3
Spinach in cream sauce with garlic and nutmeg			
for 2:	300	15	9
per serving:	150	8	5
Petit pois, carrots and babycorn			
for 2:	300	12	6
per serving:	150	6	3

Pasta and Rice

All meals containing pasta and rice must be excluded. There is an immense range of these ready-made meals available, of which the following are merely typical examples. Although some meals may not seem to contain as much carbohydrates as others (for example, beef lasagne), most of the meal consists of refined carbohydrates, which contain no essential nutrients, so there is virtually no nutrition in the meal. The aim of this diet is not only to lose excess weight but also to be healthy, and refined carbohydrates are virtually devoid of the nutrients you need for health – so eliminate them from your diet as much as possible.

Meal	Weight (g)	Carbs (g)	Protein (g)
Spaghetti Bolognaise			
for 2:	400	51	28
per serving:	200	26	14
Beef lasagne			
for 2:	380	42	22
per serving:	190	21	11
Macaroni cheese	250	31	18
Cajun chicken fettucine			
for 2:	500	65	40
per serving:	250	33	20
Chicken con carne with rice			
for 2:	500	106	30
per serving:	250	53	15
Vegetable curry			
for 2:	400	80	12
per serving:	200	40	6
Chargrilled chicken risotto			
for 2:	365	44	22
per serving:	183	22	11
Chicken linguine with salsa verde			
for 2:	400	56	28
per serving:	200	28	14

Meal	Weight (g)	Carbs (g)	Protein (g)
Tomato and Marscapone risotto			
for 2:	365	62	7
per serving:	186	31	4
Tuna and pasta bake			
for 2:	400	48	28
per serving:	200	24	14
Chicken curry			
for 2:	400	88	24
per serving:	200	44	12
Chicken fajitas with salsa and sour cream dips			
for 2:	490	80	48
per serving:	245	40	24
Haggis with potatoes and turnip			
for 2:	340	53	17
per serving:	170	27	9
Steak fajitas			
for 2:	460	83	41
per serving:	230	42	21
Sweet and sour chicken			
for 2:	300	72	21
per serving:	150	36	11
Chilli nachos			
for 2:	400	116	32
per serving:	200	58	16
Steak and kidney pie			
for 4:	620	143	87
per serving:	155	31	17

Indian meals

Unfortunately different take-away outlets vary in their preparation and contents of seemingly identical meals. Some may add carbohydrates to their recipes whereas others may not, so it's probably best to severely restrict Indian take-away meals on this diet – or simply ask whether sugar is added to a selected meal. If so, ask for this to be omitted. Indications of meals which can be safely included in the diet, providing there is no added sugar, are listed on page 236.

This does not, however, mean that Indian food is forbidden on this diet. On the contrary, there are other ways of enjoying this delicious food whilst still adhering to a low-carb diet and a hectic lifestyle. Obviously, the simplest way to enjoy the food and be sure of the exact carbohydrate content is to cook it yourself; recipes for this very purpose are described in the Quick-and-easy dinner section of the book (pages 181–218). But if you really have virtually no time – or you simply don't want to cook (or can't cook) – there is a perfect fast food alternative: microwavable ready-prepared Indian meals are widely available from supermarkets and are ready in less than 5 minutes. But, you must be careful to choose judiciously because some are very low-carb and others are very high-carb. Not for the first time in this book (and certainly not for the last) we strongly advise you to *read the label*. The nutritional content of the meal is printed on the side (or the rear) of the packaging and a quick check of the *total carbohydrate content* of the meal will instantly inform you whether you can include it in your low-carb diet or not. Incidentally, the external appearance of the packaging will give absolutely no indication whatsoever to the internal contents. The following Indian meals – all from the same outlet – have virtually identical packaging and size, yet vary from 10 grams of carbohydrate to 77 grams of carbohydrate per meal! Read the label, and you can easily differentiate between those to enjoy and those to leave on the shelf. The protein content as well as the carbohydrate content has been described for each meal to demonstrate how nutritious these meals can be.

Indian meals which can be safely included in a low-carb diet

Meal	Weight (g)	Carbs (g)	Protein (g)
Chicken korma	350	13	45
Chicken balti	350	14	38
Chicken makhani	350	24	39
Chicken sag	350	14	39
Chicken tikka masala	350	26	43
Chicken tariwala	350	16	39
Chicken kashmiri	350	24	39
Prawn piri	250	23	18
King prawn makhani	350	10	21
Lamb bhuna	350	21	37
Lamb rogan josh	350	18	45

Indian meals which must be excluded from a low-carb diet

Meal	Weight (g)	Carbs (g)	Protein (g)
Chicken biryani	400	79	31
Chicken piri piri	350	31	37
Lamb biryani	400	77	29

Other examples of Indian-style food which must be avoided include vegetable samosas (32 grams of carbohydrate per 100 grams) and onion bhajis (24 grams of carbohydrate per 100 grams). Read the label and you will keep to your diet easily and safely.

Restaurant meals

It is much easier than you would expect to keep to your low-carb diet when dining in a restaurant as most of the food is actually highly nutritious and of high quality. Obviously you have to avoid the carbohydrate 'fillers' like bread, rice, pasta, potatoes and parsnips, and, equally obviously, desserts are definitely out, but you can enjoy most of the *really* delicious food on the menu with little further restrictions. And providing you keep to dry white wine or red wine you can also enjoy 2–3 glasses of wine with no adverse effects on your diet.

Restaurants vary in their preparation of meals. If you are in any doubt whether sugar has been added to the meal, especially in the case of Chinese, Thai and Indian meals where it may be easily masked by the flavours, simply request that sugars and other non-artificial sweeteners should not be added to your meal. Most restaurants are very receptive to the varied tastes of their customers, particularly as many people have serious food allergies which may be life threatening.

With these few restrictions, the choice of meals is almost unlimited. We have provided some examples of the wide choice that is available to you on this diet but armed with the knowledge of the basic principles of the diet (coupled with a copy of the pocket-sized *The Ultimate Diet Counter*) you will have no difficulty in selecting appropriate meals from most menus.

Here are some typical examples of meals which meet all the requirements. All the menus have been obtained from restaurants in London and are representative of typical restaurant menus.

Bistro

Entrée

The following can be included in the diet:
 Broccoli soup
 Smoked eel salad, pancetta, soft boiled egg, mustard
  and horseradish
 Blue crab and avocado salad with mango
  and chilli dressing
 Ibrian black foot ham with aged Parmesan

The following can be included, omitting the carbohydrates:
 Pickled herrings, cucumber and potato salad
  Advice: leave the potatoes
 Warm vine tomato tart with lamb lettuce and opal basil
  *Advice: enjoy the tomatoes, lettuce and basil but
  leave the carbohydrate-rich tart*
 Lion of new season Welsh lamb with pink fir apple
  potatoes, maple syrup and mint dressing
  Advice: no maple syrup dressing or potatoes

Meals to be avoided:
 Smoked haddock fishcakes with aioli
  *Advice: fishcakes contain a variable amount of
  potato so are best avoided completely*

Main course

The following can be included in the diet:
 Veal topside, anchovy and sage
 Seared sesame tuna with pak choi, mirin and soy
 Scotch fillet steak carpaccio with Dijon mustard and
  horseradish

Duck breast and warm goats cheese salad with walnut vinaigrette

New season grilled artichokes with gorgonzola and rocket

Lime and chilli corn-fed chicken breast with avocado salsa

Grilled Angus fillet of beef with truffle mash and roast vine tomatoes

Field mushrooms stuffed with goats cheese, roasted with a basil crust and drizzled with a walnut dressing

The following meals can be included, omitting the carbohydrates:

Pan-fried foie gras with toasted brioche and fig chutney
Advice: leave the brioche

Lamb leg, aubergine, fennel and chickpea
Advice: leave the chickpeas

Chicken, hummus and raita
Advice: leave the hummus

Roasted rump of lamb with minted couscous and harissa
Advice: leave the couscous and harissa

Grilled haddock fillet set on a tartare potato mash with marinated cherry tomatoes, olives and sage
Advice: leave the potato mash

Roasted vegetable tartlet served on a bed of mixed leaves and masked by a tomato and tarragon sauce and topped with a sweet red onion crème fraîche
Advice: enjoy the vegetables but leave the carbohydrate tartlet

Grilled swordfish loin served on basil crusted potatoes, topped with roasted pak-choi and surrounded by capsicum and advocado salsa
Advice: once again, leave the potatoes

Pasta and rice-based dishes are excluded from the diet, so the following meals are examples of those which must be omitted:

Asparagus and thyme risotto with rocket and parmesan

Lobster and shrimp ravioli with baby leeks and shellfish and caviar bisque

Dessert

Desserts must be excluded during the weight loss phase of the diet, but you can enjoy cheese and grapes – simply avoid the crackers!

Brie de Meaux, Roquefort and Crottin de Chavignol with celery and grapes

Italian Restaurant

Obviously, pizza and pastas are excluded, but there is much more to Italian cuisine than these high-carb foods.

Entrée

The following can be included in the diet:

Seafood salad

Scallops Venetian style

Parma ham and melon

Baked artichoke

Mozzarella salad

Melon cocktail

Cozze marinara – mussels with garlic, oregano and tomato sauce

Verdura mista all griglia – grilled mixed vegetables served with virgin oil

Prosciutto e melone – Parma ham and melon

Bread is virtually pure carbohydrate, so the following meal is excluded:

Funghi Dell Ortolona – Fried Mushrooms in Breadcrumbs served with Tartare Sauce

Main course

The following can be included in the diet:
Poached salmon with asparagus
Maize-fed chicken with tomato and herbs
Selection of Italian cured meats served with grilled
pecorino
Florette of smoked salmon with marinated fennel and
sweet mustard dressing

The following can be included, omitting the carbohydrates:
Sweet herring with potato and herb salad
Advice: leave the potato
Roast partridge with polenta and black mushrooms
Advice: leave the polenta

*The following are excluded from the diet. All pasta is
excluded during the weight loss phase. Sweet and sour
sauces can be enjoyed when home-made – and you
know how much sugar is included – but are likely to
be very high in carbohydrates in a restaurant, and
should therefore be avoided.*
Lamb cutlets with a sweet and sour sauce
Penne with Luganega sausage, sun-dried tomatoes and
radicchio
Spaghetti al pomodoro – spaghetti with tomato sauce
Linguine pescatore – pasta with sea food sauce
Lasagne montanara – lasagne pasta with mixed
vegetables
Risotto mare – rice, sea food and tomato sauce
Cannelloni vegetariane – cannelloni filled with mixed
vegetables
Tagliatelle with aubergines, tomatoes and black olives

French cuisine

Entrée

The following can be included in the diet:

Moules marinières – the classic combination of steamed mussels with garlic, parsley, white wine and a dash of cream

Tartare of red mullet with vinaigrette of vine tomatoes

Mosaic of rabbit and foie gras and sauce gribiche

Warm salad of cramelised veal sweetbreads, wild mushrooms

Escargots sautés bourguignonne

Poached oysters, sabayon of champagne oscietra caviar

Les 6 escargots de Bourgogne – snails cooked with garlic and parsley butter

Carpaccio de saumon frais a l'huile d'olive et fleur de Guerande – carpaccio of fresh salmon marinated with olive oil and sea salt

Salade de tomates du chef – tomato, spring onions, coriander, olive oil and spice

Salade Bel Air – mozzarella cheese with sundried tomato, lamb's lettuce, roasted red onions, shaved Parmesan and a drizzle of balsamic vinigar

Mangue et poulet fume, mixed leaf salad with smoked chicken and mango

The following are included, omitting the carbohydrates:

Chicken liver pâté – a rich chicken liver pâté served with apple and red onion compote and toasted brioche bread
Advice: leave the brioche bread

Warm salad of smoked duck – roast slices of smoked duck with walnuts, spring onions, shredded cucumber and deep fried noodles all tossed in a spiced plum dressing
Advice: leave the noodles

Soupe a l'oignon au pot ancienne – French onion soup
served inside a cottage loaf topped with Gruyere
Advice: enjoy the soup and Gruyere cheese, but no bread

Main course

The following can be included in the diet:
Carre d'agneau persille et son poelon de legumes –
pan fried lamb, honey and lemon sauce
Carre d'agneau au romarin – roast rack of lamb with
rosemary
Cailles farcies aux raisins – two de-boned and stuffed
quails with port soaked raisins
Loup de mer, pan fried sea bass with prawns on a
bed of spinach and roasted cherry tomatoes.

The following can be included with minor amendments:
Poulet Piaf – baked chicken breast served on a
creamy mashed potato with mushroom, tarragon
and cream sauce
Advice: leave the mashed potato
Lamb shank – lamb on the bone braised until tender
with wine and root vegetables and served with
mashed potatoes, with a rich red wine sauce
Advice: once again, leave the mashed potato
Grilled vegetables with couscous – aubergine, sweet
pepper and courgettes on tomato couscous, topped
with fried haloumi cheese and drizzled with
vinaigrette.
Advice: leave the high-carb couscous
Steak frites et salade – the traditional Bouchon's
steak, French fries and salad
Advice: fairly obvious, leave the French fries
Medallions de lotte a l'ancienne accompagnes de son
flan de courgette – sliced monkfish served with
courgette flan
Advice: enjoy the courgettes but leave the flan

Tartiflette avec saucisses de Cumberland –
  Cumberland sausages with tartiflette (creamy
  layered potato and chopped bacon)
  Advice: leave the potatoes

Chinese Restaurants

Once again, avoid rice, sweet-and-sour dishes and meals
with batter, and most of the remainder of the menu
can be safely incorporated in the diet. But definitely no
fishcakes (which are often potato cakes in disguise!).

Entrée

The following can be included in the diet:
Stir-fried minced pork with garlic and pepper
  wrapped in a lettuce leaf
Beef in chilli bean oil with chillies and sweet basil
Pork with garlic and pepper
Mixed vegetables with mushroom sauce
Roasted baby squid with garlic and chilli deep fried
  with garlic and peppercorn salt
Aubergine and asparagus
Jelly fish with cucumber
Shark fin soup
Spicy beef shin

*The following are high-carb and definitely excluded
from the diet:*
Vegetable spring rolls
Red snapper fish cake
King prawns in tempura flour served with sweet chilli
  sauce

Main course

The following may be included in your diet:
Drunken chicken
Stuffed crab claws

Mixed vegetables (minced) lettuce wrap
Aromatic crispy duck
Lobster with stir-fried vegetables
Seabass steamed with shredded pork, chinese
   mushroom, spring onion and soya sauce
Beef in oyster sauce
Crab with pak choi
Roasted crispy chicken (Cantonese)
Stir-fried mixed vegetables
Pak choy with garlic sauce
King prawn with two kind of mushrooms
Curry chicken

*The following are high-carb and must be excluded
from the diet:*
Sesame prawn toast
Phoenix king prawns with batter
Deep fried won ton, sweet and sour dip
Sweet and sour pork
Crispy minced bean curd stewed in oyster sauce

Indian Restaurants

The high-carbohydrate components of Indian meals are
obvious: avoid rice, all forms of bread (such as naan,
chapattis and popadoms), meals with pulses (such as
dahl) and all deep-fried carbohydrates (such as pakoras
and samosas).

Entrée

The following can be included in the diet:
Prawns on puree
Murg kebab, chicken minced with onions, special
   herbs and spices
Galouti kebab
Saffron infused chargrilled scallops served in a
   creamy sauce
Baked aubergine steaks with assorted side dishes

The following must be excluded from the diet:

Raja prawn pakora

Kaju and peas samosa

Samosa, pancakes filled with spicy mincemeat and deep fried Onion bhajias

Chicken drumsticks marinated in a South Indian masala, coated with a spiced gramflour batter

Deep fried Samundri – squid rings, mussels, king prawn and whitebait coated with spiced semolina, crisp fried and served with mint chutney

Vegetable samosas

Main course

The following can be included in the diet:

Escalopes of chicken breast cooked in rich saffron-flavoured sauce

Tiger prawns marinated in ginger, yoghurt, chilli oil and spices

Vension cutlets with mustard oil, homemade Indian five spice, roast garlic and button onions

Chicken tandoori

Lamb tandoori

Murgh peshawar

Lamb peshawar

Meat kofta

Lamb rogan josh

Chicken korma

Lamb korma

Keema korma

Prawn madras

Balti chicken

Balti lamb

Shah gostaba, lamb flavoured with mild Kasmiri herbs, cooked in fresh cream

Rogon chicken, medium cooked with tomatoes

Vegetable curry cooked with special spices

Succulent chicken breast dices marinated in a
  classical yoghurt and spice mixture
A Moghal chicken korma in a rich and creamy
  sauce made from cashew nuts and poppy seeds

Thai restaurants

Entrée

The following can be included in the diet:
Thai seafood platter
Marinated chicken with peanut sauce on skewers
Tiger prawns
Mussels in special sauce

The following are definitely excluded from the diet:
Vegetable spring rolls
Spicy corn cake with curry paste
Minced pork/prawn on toast
Spicy thai fishcake served with cucumber and nut
  pickle

Main course

*The following can be included in your diet, obviously
excluding any rice side-dishes:*
Green curry with beef, chicken or prawns thai
  Muslim beef curry
Roasted duck curry
Stir-fried beef, chicken or prawns
Grilled whole spring chicken
Stir-fried aubergine, chilli and basil
Beansprouts, stir-fried with spring onions

Dessert

All desserts are completely excluded during the weight loss phase of the diet. Here are a few typical examples of very high-carb desserts:

Bitter chocolate tart with white chocolate mousse
Passion fruit crème brulée
Lemon tart with lime crème fraîche
Fresh fruit salad with organic vanilla and honey ice-cream
Chocolate and raspberry tart with clotted cream and fresh berries
Callestik farm ice-cream
Tiramisu, surrounded by a Marsala crème anglaise
Traditional Thai sweet
Fried banana fritters
Sorbet (various)
Ice-cream

Chapter 8

Vegetables and Salads

Vegetable side-dishes

Chilli vegetables   253–54
Basil Bocconcini with spinach   254–55
Hoisin vegetables   255–56
Peperonata   256
Teriyaki tofu   256–57
Pepper and herb frittata   257–58
Stir-fried vegetables with black bean
    sauce   258
Bok choi with cinnamon   259
Spinach with butter sauce   259
Asparagus with wild rocket and mint
    sauce   260
Brussels sprouts with orange and lemon
    butter sauce   260–61
Broccoli with garlic and spring onions   261
Watercress with ginger   261–62
Cherry tomatoes with basil and
    coriander   262
Baby leeks in lemon butter sauce   262–63

Salads

Crispy herb salad   263
Tikka masala salad   263–64
Three-cheese salad   264
Radish and mint salad   265
Chicken and wild rocket salad   265–66
Rocket and tofu salad   266
Radicchio and cucumber salad   267
Gazpacho salad   267–68

Vegetable side-dishes

Fresh vegetables are an essential part of any healthy diet. However, the problem for busy people is that they seem to be too time-consuming, both in preparation and cooking. This need not be the case. As already explained, fresh vegetables can be purchased ready-prepared: mangetout, French beans, carrots julienne, broccoli florets, peas, asparagus, spinach, sugarsnap peas and cauliflower florets – to name a few – are all instantly available for cooking. By steaming or microwaving fresh vegetables they can be ready in minutes, will retain almost all their healthy nutrients and cook without supervision. So there really is no reason why everyone, irrespective of how busy they may be, cannot enjoy delicious and healthy vegetables as an integral part of a healthy diet. Of course, vegetables alone are rather bland so we have added quick and easy flavours and sauces which complement the vegetables perfectly.

Chilli vegetables

For 2

2 tbsp extra-virgin olive oil
1 medium red onion, peeled and chopped
1 garlic clove, peeled and chopped
1 medium red pepper, deseeded and sliced

1 medium yellow pepper, deseeded and sliced
50 grams mangetout
1 tbsp Sharwood's hot chilli sauce

- Heat the extra-virgin olive oil in a wok.
- Sauté the onion and garlic for 1–2 minutes
- Stir in the peppers and mangetout and stir-fry for 2–3 minutes
- Stir in the chilli sauce, simmer for 1-2 minutes and serve immediately.

CARBOHYDRATE CONTENT PER SERVING: 12 GRAMS

Quick method

For 2
2 tbsp extra-virgin olive oil
250-gram bag pre-chopped stir-fry vegetables
1 tbsp Sharwood's hot chilli sauce

- Heat the extra-virgin olive oil in a wok.
- Stir-fry the vegetables for 2–3 minutes.
- Stir in the chilli sauce, simmer for 1–2 minutes and serve immediately.

CARBOHYDRATE CONTENT PER SERVING: 5 GRAMS

Basil Bocconcini with spinach

For 2
2 tbsp extra-virgin olive oil
1 medium red onion, peeled and chopped
1 garlic clove, peeled and finely chopped
200 grams fresh spinach, stalks removed
freshly ground black pepper
1 tbsp chopped fresh basil leaves
3 large free-range eggs, beaten
125 grams Bocconcini cheese, thinly sliced

- Heat the extra-virgin olive oil in a medium frying pan and sauté the onion and garlic for 1–2 minutes.
- Add the spinach and gently stir-fry for 2–3 minutes.
- Season to taste, remove from the heat and allow to cool.
- Mix the spinach mixture with the basil and eggs, and pour the mixture into an oven-safe baking dish.
- Top with a layer of sliced Bocconcini and cover with pierced aluminium foil.
- Cook in the centre of a pre-heated oven at 180°C (gas 4) for 20–25 minutes and serve immediately.

CARBOHYDRATE CONTENT PER SERVING: 7 GRAMS

Hoisin vegetables

A delicious accompaniment to many meals.

For 2
2 tbsp extra-virgin olive oil
4 spring onions, chopped on the diagonal into 3–4 cm lengths
1 garlic clove, peeled and chopped
4 slices fresh root ginger, peeled and chopped
3 medium courgettes, sliced lengthways
1 medium red pepper, deseeded and sliced
1 medium yellow pepper, deseeded and sliced
2 tbsp hoisin sauce
freshly ground black pepper

- Heat the extra-virgin olive oil in a wok and stir-fry the spring onions, garlic, ginger, courgettes and peppers for 3–4 minutes.
- Add the hoisin sauce and stir-fry for a further 2–3 minutes, season to taste and serve immediately.

CARBOHYDRATE CONTENT PER SERVING: 16 GRAMS

Peperonata

For 4
3 tbsp extra-virgin olive oil
1 large red onion, peeled and chopped
1 garlic clove, peeled and finely chopped
4 medium red peppers, deseeded and finely sliced
400-gram tin plum tomatoes
1 tbsp chopped fresh basil (or 1 tsp dried basil)
1 tbsp chopped fresh parsley (optional)
freshly ground black pepper

- Heat the extra-virgin olive oil in a medium frying pan and sauté the onion and garlic for 1–2 minutes.
- Stir in the peppers and stir-fry for a further 3–4 minutes.
- Drain the tomatoes.
- Add the tomatoes, basil and parsley, and simmer gently over a low heat for 3–4 minutes.
- Season to taste and serve immediately.

CARBOHYDRATE CONTENT PER SERVING: 10 GRAMS

Teriyaki tofu

This meal should be prepared the evening before use – if possible – to allow the tofu to marinate. Preparation time is minimal and the meal is ready immediately the following day.

For 2

80 grams tofu, cubed
2 tbsp sake
2 tbsp mirin (sweet rice wine)
2 tbsp shoyu (Japanese soy sauce)
2 slices fresh root ginger, peeled and finely chopped
2 spring onions, finely chopped

- Mix together the tofu, sake, mirin, shoyu, ginger root and spring onions and marinate in the fridge for 24 hours.
- Serve the following day.

CARBOHYDRATE CONTENT PER SERVING: 3 GRAMS

Pepper and herb frittata

For 2

2 tbsp extra-virgin olive oil
1 small orange pepper, deseeded and diced
1 small green pepper, deseeded and diced
3 spring onions, chopped into 2 cm lengths on the diagonal
4 large free-range eggs, beaten
50 ml full-cream milk
1 tbsp chopped fresh mint leaves
1 tbsp chopped fresh coriander leaves
100 grams Edam cheese, grated
freshly ground black pepper

- Heat the extra-virgin olive oil in a medium frying pan and sauté the peppers and spring onions for 2–3 minutes.
- Mix the beaten eggs with the milk and add to the pan, stirring gently.
- Cook over a medium heat for 2–3 minutes.
- Sprinkle over the chopped mint and coriander, and top with grated cheese.

257

- Grill under a hot grill, no closer than 8–10 cm from the grill, until the cheese begins to bubble.
- Season to taste and serve immediately.

CARBOHYDRATE CONTENT PER SERVING: 7 GRAMS

Stir-fried vegetables with black bean sauce

For 2

2 tbsp extra-virgin olive oil
4 spring onions, chopped on the diagonal
1 garlic clove, peeled and chopped
3 slices fresh root ginger, peeled and chopped
75 grams chestnut mushrooms, wiped and halved lengthways
75 grams beansprouts
75 grams mangetout
1 medium red pepper, deseeded and sliced
freshly ground black pepper

Sauce

2 tsp cornflour
4 tbsp water
2 tbsp dry sherry
1 tbsp light soy sauce
2 tbsp black bean sauce

- To make the sauce, stir the cornflour into the water in a small bowl, then stir in the other ingredients for the sauce.
- Heat the extra-virgin olive oil in a wok and stir-fry the spring onions, garlic, ginger, mushrooms, beansprouts, mangetout and pepper for 2–3 minutes.
- Add the sauce and stir-fry for a further 3–4 minutes.
- Season to taste and serve immediately.

CARBOHYDRATE CONTENT PER SERVING: 15 GRAMS

Bok choi with cinnamon

For 2
1 medium bok choi, chopped
½ tsp ground cinnamon

- Place the bok choi halves in a steamer and lightly-steam for 4–5 minutes.

Or
- Place the bok choi in a microwave-safe container, add 1 tablespoon of water, cover and cook on 'high' for about 3 minutes. Allow to stand for 1 minute.

- Sprinkle over the ground cinnamon and serve immediately.

CARBOHYDRATE CONTENT PER SERVING: 1 GRAM

Spinach with butter sauce

For 2
50 grams unsalted butter
1 garlic clove, peeled and finely chopped
100 grams fresh spinach leaves
freshly ground black pepper

- Heat the butter in a medium saucepan and sauté the garlic for about a minute.
- Stir in the spinach leaves and toss the leaves in the melted butter.
- Stir frequently until the spinach leaves begin to soften, usually 1–2 minutes. Be careful not to overcook otherwise the spinach leaves can wilt and virtually disappear in a matter of seconds!
- Season to taste and serve immediately.

CARBOHYDRATE CONTENT PER SERVING: 1 GRAM

Asparagus with wild rocket and mint sauce

For 2
100 grams asparagus, washed and trimmed
wild rocket and mint sauce (page 276)
lemon wedges, to garnish

- Place the asparagus in the base of a suitable microwave-safe container, arranging the thick stalks to the outside of the dish and the thin tops facing inwards.
- Add 2 tablespoons water, cover and cook on 'high' for 2½–3 minutes, then allow to stand for 1 minute.

Or
- Lightly steam the asparagus for 10–12 minutes.

At the same time
- Prepare the rocket and mint sauce.

- Serve the asparagus, drizzle over the lemon juice and top with rocket and mint sauce.

CARBOHYDRATE CONTENT PER SERVING: 4 GRAMS

Brussels sprouts with orange and lemon butter sauce

For 2
100 grams Brussels sprouts
50 grams butter
1 tbsp freshly squeezed orange juice
1 tbsp freshly squeezed lemon juice
1 tsp chopped fresh mint leaves (optional)

- Remove the outer leaves of the Brussels sprouts, trim the base and score the base with a cross.
- Place the Brussels sprouts in a microwave-safe container, add 2 tablespoons of water, cover and

cook on 'high' for 2½–3 minutes, then allow to stand for 1 minute.

Or
- Lightly steam the Brussels sprouts for 15 minutes.

At the same time
- Heat the butter in a small saucepan and stir in the orange and lemon juice.
- Pour the citrus butter over the Brussels sprouts and sprinkle with chopped fresh mint leaves.

CARBOHYDRATE CONTENT PER SERVING: 3 GRAMS

Broccoli with garlic and spring onions

For 2
2 tbsp extra-virgin olive oil
75 grams broccoli florets
1 garlic clove, peeled and finely chopped
3 spring onions, chopped into 3–4 cm lengths on the diagonal
freshly ground black pepper

- Heat the extra-virgin olive oil in a wok and stir-fry the broccoli, garlic and spring onions for 3–4 minutes.
- Season to taste with freshly ground black pepper and serve immediately.

CARBOHYDRATE CONTENT PER SERVING: 2 GRAMS

Watercress with ginger

For 2
50 grams unsalted butter
150 grams watercress
2 slices fresh root ginger, peeled and finely chopped
freshly ground black pepper

- Heat the butter in a medium saucepan and add the watercress and ginger.
- Stir frequently to coat the watercress evenly.
- Remove from the heat as soon as the watercress begins to soften, season to taste and serve immediately.

CARBOHYDRATE CONTENT PER SERVING: 2 GRAMS

Cherry tomatoes with basil and coriander

For 2
50 grams unsalted butter
10 cherry vine tomatoes
1 tsp chopped fresh basil
1 tsp chopped fresh coriander
freshly ground black pepper

- Heat the butter in a medium saucepan, add the cherry tomatoes, basil and coriander and sauté for 2–3 minutes.
- Season to taste with freshly ground black pepper and serve immediately.

CARBOHYDRATE CONTENT PER SERVING: 4 GRAMS

Baby leeks in lemon butter sauce

For 2
6 baby leeks
50 grams unsalted butter
3 tbsp freshly squeezed lemon juice

- Place the baby leeks in a microwave-safe container, add 2 tablespoons water, cover and microwave on 'high' for 3 minutes.

Or

- Lightly steam the baby leeks for about 10 minutes.

At the same time
- Melt the butter in a small saucepan, stir in the lemon juice and heat through gently for about a minute.
- Serve the leeks and pour over the lemon butter sauce.

CARBOHYDRATE CONTENT PER SERVING: 2 GRAMS

Salads

In addition to the following, salad recipes are described on pages 40–41, and of course there are many alternative salad recipes in *The New High Protein Diet* and *The New High Protein Diet Cookbook*.

Crispy herb salad

For 2
100 grams mixed green salad leaves (rocket, coral, watercress, green oak, mizuna and frisée)
1 tbsp chopped fresh flat-leaf parsley
1 tbsp chopped fresh mint
1 tbsp chopped fresh basil
freshly ground black pepper
vinaigrette, home-made (pages 273–74) or commercial

- Mix together the green salad leaves, flat-leaf parsley, mint and basil, and season to taste.
- Drizzle over the vinaigrette of choice.

CARBOHYDRATE CONTENT PER SERVING: 3 GRAMS

Tikka masala salad

For 2
2 tbsp extra-virgin olive oil
150g turkey breast, sliced into thin strips
100 ml commercial tikka sauce
¼ English cucumber, chopped
2 medium vine-ripened plum tomatoes, chopped

2 tsp chopped fresh mint leaves
1 tbsp mayonnaise
freshly ground black pepper

- Heat the extra-virgin olive oil in a wok and stir-fry the turkey breast for 3–4 minutes.
- Stir in the tikka sauce and set aside to cool.
- Mix together the cucumber, tomatoes, mint and mayonnaise in a medium bowl.
- Serve with the tikka turkey breast and season to taste.

CARBOHYDRATE CONTENT PER SERVING: 7 GRAMS

Three-cheese salad

For 2

50 grams mozzarella cheese, sliced
50 grams Emmental cheese, cubed
8 cherry vine tomatoes, halved
2 spring onions, chopped into 3–4 cm lengths on the diagonal
8 black olives, stoned and halved
75 grams crispy green lettuce leaves (mizuna, frisée, green oak and cos)
30 grams Parmesan cheese, grated
drizzle of balsamic vinaigrette
freshly ground black pepper

- Mix together the mozzarella cheese, Emmental cheese, cherry tomatoes, spring onions, olives and crispy green lettuce leaves in a large salad bowl.
- Sprinkle over the grated Parmesan, drizzle over some balsamic vinaigrette and season to taste.
- Serve immediately.

CARBOHYDRATE CONTENT PER SERVING: 5 GRAMS

Radish and mint salad

For 2

6 cherry vine tomatoes, halved
4 radishes, thinly sliced
1 tbsp chopped fresh mint leaves
1 tbsp chopped fresh chives
1 celery stick, chopped on the diagonal
1 small Hass avocado, stone removed, peeled and diced
150 ml crème fraîche
freshly ground black pepper
75 grams wild rocket leaves

- Mix together the tomatoes, radishes, mint, chives, celery and avocado in a medium bowl, then stir in the crème fraîche.
- Lay a bed of wild rocket leaves on each plate, top with the radish crème fraîche mixture and season to taste with freshly ground black pepper.
- Serve immediately.

CARBOHYDRATE CONTENT PER SERVING: 9 GRAMS

Chicken and wild rocket salad

For 2

2 chicken breasts approximately 125–150 grams each
30 grams unsalted butter
6 cherry vine tomatoes, halved
1 medium Hass avocado, peeled, stone removed and chopped
1 tbsp chopped fresh coriander
1 tbsp chopped fresh chives
75 grams wild rocket leaves
drizzle of French vinaigrette
freshly ground black pepper

- Place the chicken breasts in an oven-safe dish and dot with butter.

- Cover with pierced aluminium foil and cook in the centre of a pre-heated oven at 180°C (gas 4) for 35–40 minutes, then set aside to cool.

Or
- Use two chicken breasts which have been purchased ready-cooked.
- Chop the chicken breast into cubes.
- Mix together the chicken breast, tomatoes, avocado, coriander, chives and wild rocket in a large salad bowl, drizzle over some French vinaigrette and season to taste with freshly ground black pepper.
- Serve immediately.

CARBOHYDRATE CONTENT PER SERVING: 6 GRAMS

Rocket and tofu salad

For 2
1 tbsp sesame seeds
100 grams tofu, chopped into small cubes
100 grams mixed rocket and wild rocket leaves
1 small red pepper, deseeded and thinly sliced
1 small yellow pepper, deseeded and thinly sliced
75 ml lemon vinaigrette, home-made (page 274) or commercial
freshly ground black pepper
sprigs of fresh mint, to garnish (optional)

- Place the sesame seeds in a small frying pan and dry-fry for 1–2 minutes.
- Mix together the sesame seeds, tofu, rocket and peppers in a medium salad bowl.
- Drizzle over the lemon vinaigrette and season to taste with freshly ground black pepper.
- Garnish with sprigs of fresh mint.

CARBOHYDRATE CONTENT PER SERVING: 6 GRAMS

Radicchio and cucumber salad

For 2

2 Lebanese cucumbers, sliced vertically into thin
  strips
3 large plum tomatoes, sliced
1 tsp capers, rinsed
1 tbsp cashew nuts
1 tbsp chopped fresh chives
1 medium radicchio lettuce, leaves separated
2 tbsp balsamic vinaigrette
freshly ground black pepper

- Mix together the sliced cucumber, tomatoes, capers,
  cashew nuts and chives in a medium bowl.
- Place a bed of radicchio lettuce on each plate and
  top with the salad mixture.
- Drizzle over a little balsamic vinaigrette and
  season to taste with freshly ground black pepper.

CARBOHYDRATE CONTENT PER SERVING: 9 GRAMS

Gazpacho salad

For 2

1 small green pepper, deseeded and thinly sliced
1 small red pepper, deseeded and thinly sliced
1 small yellow pepper, deseeded and thinly sliced
8 small Pomodorino plum tomatoes, halved vertically
2 spring onions, finely chopped
1 Lebanese cucumber, diced
1 tbsp chopped fresh flat-leaf parsley
drizzle of French vinaigrette, home-made (page 273)
  or commercial
freshly ground black pepper

- Mix together the sliced peppers, tomatoes, spring
  onions, cucumber and parsley in a medium salad
  bowl.

- Drizzle over the vinaigrette of choice and season to taste with freshly ground black pepper.
- Serve immediately.

CARBOHYDRATE CONTENT PER SERVING: 9 GRAMS

Chapter 9

Dressings and Sauces

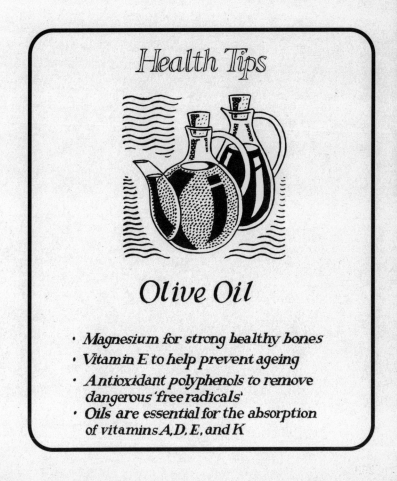

Health Tips

Olive Oil

- *Magnesium for strong healthy bones*
- *Vitamin E to help prevent ageing*
- *Antioxidant polyphenols to remove dangerous 'free radicals'*
- *Oils are essential for the absorption of vitamins A, D, E, and K*

French vinaigrette   273
Balsamic vinaigrette   274
Lemon vinaigrette   274
Tomato sauce   274–75
Basil pesto sauce   275
Mango raita   275
Cucumber raita   276
Wild rocket and mint sauce   276

The preparation of dressings and sauces is not a 'normal' pastime for most busy people with a hectic lifestyle, however it is important to realise how quick, easy and healthy it is to prepare a few dressings and sauces – and now incredibly economical when compared to commercial varieties. Here are a few very simple examples which literally anyone can prepare in a few minutes although many more are described in *The New High Protein Diet* and *The New High Protein Diet Cookbook*.

The quantities of vinaigrettes have been deliberately increased; vinaigrette will easily store in the fridge and the amount of effort to produce eight servings (i.e. four meals for two people) is effectively the same as the amount of effort to produce two servings.

French vinaigrette

For 8
250 ml extra-virgin olive oil
75 ml white wine vinegar
2 tsp dry mustard powder
1 large garlic clove, peeled and grated
freshly ground black pepper

- Put the ingredients of the vinaigrette in a large screw-top jar and shake vigorously to mix.

CARBOHYDRATE CONTENT PER SERVING: < 1 GRAM

Balsamic vinaigrette

For 8
250 ml extra-virgin olive oil
75 ml balsamic vinegar
1 large garlic clove, peeled and grated
freshly ground black pepper

- Add the ingredients of the vinaigrette to a large
  screw-top jar and shake vigorously to mix.

CARBOHYDRATE CONTENT PER SERVING: 2 GRAMS

Lemon vinaigrette

For 8
250 ml extra-virgin olive oil
60 ml freshly squeezed lemon juice
freshly ground black pepper

- Add the ingredients of the vinaigrette to a large
  screw-top jar and shake vigorously to mix.

CARBOHYDRATE CONTENT PER SERVING: <1 GRAM

Tomato sauce

For 4
400-gram tin peeled plum tomatoes
1 tbsp tomato purée
1 tsp granulated sugar
1 tbsp chopped fresh basil, or 1 tsp dried basil (optional)
freshly ground black pepper
dash of Worcestershire sauce

- Drain the tomatoes and pour into a small saucepan.
- Stir in the tomato purée, sugar and herbs, and
  season to taste.
- Return 1 tablespoon of tomato juice to the pan and

bring to a gentle simmer for 5 minutes. Cool the sauce before using.
- Add a dash of Worcestershire sauce to the remaining tomato juice and drink – enjoy!

CARBOHYDRATE CONTENT PER SERVING: 6 GRAMS

Basil pesto sauce

For 8
100 grams pine nuts
150 grams chopped fresh basil leaves
2 garlic cloves, peeled
100 grams Parmesan cheese, grated
freshly ground black pepper
150 ml extra-virgin olive oil

- Dry-fry the pine nuts for 1–2 minutes.
- Blend the pine nuts, basil, garlic, Parmesan cheese and pepper in a blender or food processor.
- Gradually add the extra-virgin olive oil whilst blending.

CARBOHYDRATE CONTENT PER SERVING: 2 GRAMS

Mango raita

For 2
100 ml natural yoghurt
¼ medium cucumber, peeled and diced
2 tsp chopped fresh coriander
¼ mango, diced
fresh mint leaves, to garnish

- Blend together the yoghurt, cucumber, coriander and mango, then set aside to cool in the fridge for at least 20 minutes.
- Garnish with fresh mint leaves and serve immediately.

CARBOHYDRATE CONTENT PER SERVING: 11 GRAMS

Cucumber raita

200 ml natural yoghurt
1 tbsp chopped fresh mint
½ tsp ground cumin
1 small Lebanese cucumber, diced

- Mix together the yoghurt, mint, cumin and cucumber in a small bowl, cover and cool in the fridge.

CARBOHYDRATE CONTENT PER SERVING: 6 GRAMS

Wild rocket and mint sauce

For 2
75 ml soured cream
1 tbsp chopped fresh wild rocket leaves
1 tbsp chopped fresh mint leaves
pinch of cayenne pepper

- Mix together the soured cream, chopped rocket and mint leaves and cayenne pepper in a medium bowl.
- Cover and cool in the fridge for 20–30 minutes before use, if possible.

CARBOHYDRATE CONTENT PER SERVING: 2 GRAMS

Chapter 10

One Month Meal Plan

Obviously it is impossible to provide a meal plan which will suit everyone because the aim of this book is to try to cater for all possible different tastes and hectic lifestyles, so we have provided a meal plan which incorporates a little of all the different lifestyles. This is only intended as an example of how versatile the diet can be, and easily adapted to the busiest of lifestyles. Some of the recipes mentioned are described in *The New High Protein Diet* and *The New High Protein Diet Cookbook*.

Week 1
Monday

Breakfast	Avocado on toast
Lunch	Roast beef salad open sandwich
Dinner	Rocket and tofu salad

TOTAL DAILY CARBOHYDRATES: 42 GRAMS

Tuesday

Breakfast	Continental breakfast
Lunch	Salmon with crème fraîche salad lunchbox
Dinner	Chilli con carne

TOTAL DAILY CARBOHYDRATES: 26 GRAMS

Wednesday

Breakfast	Poached eggs with tomatoes
Lunch	Smoked trout with avocado
Dinner	Spicy chicken drumsticks

TOTAL DAILY CARBOHYDRATES: 19 GRAMS

Thursday

Breakfast	Kippers
Lunch	Avocado and Bocconcini salad lunchbox
Dinner	Steak with spinach and caramelised onions

TOTAL DAILY CARBOHYDRATES: 14 GRAMS

Friday

Breakfast	Mushrooms with bacon
Lunch	Gammon with Balsamic vinegar
Dinner	Salmon with lime butter sauce and watercress

TOTAL DAILY CARBOHYDRATES: 11 GRAMS

Saturday

Breakfast	Continental breakfast
Lunch	Lamb cutlets with herb butter sauce
Dinner	Beef jalfrezi curry with peppers

TOTAL DAILY CARBOHYDRATES: 21 GRAMS

Sunday

Breakfast	Bacon and eggs with mushrooms and tomatoes
Lunch	Roast beef with gravy and vegetables
Dinner	Peppered smoked mackerel with spinach

TOTAL DAILY CARBOHYDRATES: 17 GRAMS

Week 2
Monday

Breakfast	Poached eggs on toast

Lunch	Chicken with mayonnaise and avocado salad lunchbox
Dinner	Beef bolognaise with mushrooms

TOTAL DAILY CARBOHYDRATES: 30 GRAMS

Tuesday

Breakfast	Whiting with herbs
Lunch	Hoisin duck crêpes
Dinner	Prawn omelette

TOTAL DAILY CARBOHYDRATES: 28 GRAMS

Wednesday

Breakfast	Continental breakfast
Lunch	Roast ham with Emmental cheese and mustard lunchbox
Dinner	Tikka masala salad

TOTAL DAILY CARBOHYDRATES: 10 GRAMS

Thursday

Breakfast	Cheese on toast with Worcestershire sauce
Lunch	Prawn mayonnaise open sandwich
Dinner	Duck with plum sauce

TOTAL DAILY CARBOHYDRATES: 48 GRAMS

Friday

Breakfast	Scrambled eggs with Parma ham
Lunch	Hot and spicy chicken drumsticks with baby spinach
Dinner	Caponata

TOTAL DAILY CARBOHYDRATES: 18 GRAMS

Saturday

Breakfast	Continental breakfast
Lunch	Shellfish with bok choy
Dinner	Turkey teriyaki

TOTAL DAILY CARBOHYDRATES: 12 GRAMS

Sunday

Breakfast	Omelette with smoked salmon and dill
Lunch	Roast pork with apple sauce and vegetables
Dinner	Peppered smoked ham with spinach and ricotta

TOTAL DAILY CARBOHYDRATES: 19 GRAMS

Week 3
Monday

Breakfast	Avocado on toast
Lunch	Prawn mayonnaise salad lunchbox
Dinner	Lamb tikka masala with broccoli

TOTAL DAILY CARBOHYDRATES: 33 GRAMS

Tuesday

Breakfast	Smoked haddock with Leerdammer cheese
Lunch	Greek salad
Dinner	Balti chicken

TOTAL DAILY CARBOHYDRATES: 11 GRAMS

Wednesday

Breakfast	Continental breakfast
Lunch	Ham, egg and chives open sandwich

Dinner	Sesame beef with ginger and lemongrass

TOTAL DAILY CARBOHYDRATES: 30 GRAMS

Thursday

Breakfast	Gammon steak and mushrooms
Lunch	Spicy prawns with rocket
Dinner	Chicken and wild rocket salad

TOTAL DAILY CARBOHYDRATES: 12 GRAMS

Friday

Breakfast	Scrambled eggs with tomatoes and basil
Lunch	Salmon with crème fraîche and salad lunchbox
Dinner	Sweet and sour beef with mangetout

TOTAL DAILY CARBOHYDRATES: 26 GRAMS

Saturday

Breakfast	Continental breakfast
Lunch	Peperonata
Dinner	Thai chicken with lemongrass and ginger

TOTAL DAILY CARBOHYDRATES: 29 GRAMS

Sunday

Breakfast	Ham and eggs
Lunch	Roast lamb with mint sauce and vegetables
Dinner	Gazpacho salad

TOTAL DAILY CARBOHYDRATES: 20 GRAMS

Week 4
Monday
Breakfast	Kippers with tomatoes
Lunch	Tuna mayonnaise open sandwich
Dinner	Chicken korma with mangetout and broccoli

TOTAL DAILY CARBOHYDRATES: 33 GRAMS

Tuesday
Breakfast	Cheese on toast with mixed herbs
Lunch	Greek salad lunchbox
Dinner	Peking duck

TOTAL DAILY CARBOHYDRATES: 31 GRAMS

Wednesday
Breakfast	Boiled eggs
Lunch	Chargrilled curry sardines with crème fraîche
Dinner	Meatballs with tomato and basil sauce

TOTAL DAILY CARBOHYDRATES: 18 GRAMS

Thursday
Breakfast	Continental breakfast
Lunch	Salami salad sandwich
Dinner	Salmon with Bocconcini and basil

TOTAL DAILY CARBOHYDRATES: 23 GRAMS

Friday
Breakfast	Tomatoes on toast with basil and coriander
Lunch	Tiger prawns with chilli and coriander vinaigrette and salad lunchbox

Dinner   Turkey in cherry tomato and
chilli sauce

TOTAL DAILY CARBOHYDRATES: 32 GRAMS

Saturday
Breakfast   Bacon and eggs with mushrooms
Lunch   Gazpacho salad
Dinner   Plaice with olives

TOTAL DAILY CARBOHYDRATES: 18 GRAMS

Sunday
Breakfast   Continental breakfast
Lunch   Moussaka
Dinner   Chicken satay with lime

TOTAL DAILY CARBOHYDRATES: 36 GRAMS

Chapter 11

Exercise Anywhere!
The 5-Minute-a-Day Plan

You don't have to exercise to diet successfully and lose body fat, but you do have to exercise if you want to be *really* healthy. Why? Because moderate exercise stimulates respiration (breathing) and improves the circulation, improving the oxygen supply to our muscles (including the heart muscle).

Moderate exercise does not involve jogging, gym training, aerobics or any of the other popular exercise regimes which come-and-go without seeming to make any significant impact on the general health of the population. The reason these exercise programmes are only successful for the fortunate few is because they are really not practical and unless you are totally committed to an exercise regime of this nature you will inevitably default and give up after a short time. This is not a personal opinion, it is an established fact with which most dieters would agree. If you require any further proof, just examine the constant turnover of most gym memberships!

Severe exercise of this nature is seldom successful as part of a weight-loss programme because *it doesn't make sense medically*. When you exercise strenuously you become very hungry. Unless you have an iron will, you must inevitably eat – usually much more than the calories you have lost in exercise. And exercise stimulates insulin production, which, as you have seen, converts excess calories to instant body fat!

Surely the logical conclusion of this reasoned argument is that exercise must be detrimental to your health. Certainly not, but the forms of *strenuous* exercise which have been described probably are not conducive to good health. Jogging places considerable stress on knees and ankles – usually on knees and ankles which have had very little exercise for many years! The commonest form of arthritis – osteoarthritis – results from a loss of cartilage from joints, essentially a form of 'wearing away' of the inner surfaces of the joint. One cannot help believe that the constant severe impact on joints, which is an inevitable consequence of jogging, must accelerate the arthritic process.

Weight training in the gym and aerobics are similarly nonsensical exercises for overweight people. When you haven't exercised to any significant degree for years you are quite simply 'out of condition'. What exactly does this mean? Your muscles have wasted so you tire easily, your respiratory function (breathing) cannot cope with excessive exertion and your cardiovascular function (heart and circulation) cannot increase sufficiently to compensate for the massive demands suddenly being placed on the muscles which require oxygen during exercise – fast! The result for the out-of-condition overweight individual who embarks upon such a sudden crash programme to lose weight as quickly as possible by unaccustomed exercise is at best physical exhaustion and pain, and at worst coronary thrombosis and early demise! It seems melodramatic but it's not. There are too many examples of heart attacks during unaccustomed exercise.

So how can exercise be healthy but also be dangerous? The obvious answer is that the *correct* form of exercise is healthy and the *wrong* form of exercise is dangerous.

The correct form of exercise will stimulate blood flow, increasing the rate of oxygen delivery to the muscles but not to extreme levels which cause pain and danger. Incidentally, pain during exercise is a danger signal. It is a warning that there is a build-up of lactic acid in the muscles which is the body's method of warning you that the muscles are not obtaining sufficient oxygen. If you continue to try to break through the pain barrier you are increasingly likely to place your life in danger. The maxim 'no pain, no gain' only applies to extremely fit athletes with a healthy heart and circulation. For the rest of us, it is a maxim for an early myocardial infarction!

The correct form of exercise for unfit people is *walking*. Yes, it is as simple as that! Walking 15-20 minutes per day is medically proven to significantly improve fitness levels. Why? Because walking increases the blood flow to the muscles, improving circulation and heart function. It also dramatically improves respiratory function (breathing) by opening up the small alveoli in the lungs. And moderate walking per day has no dangerous or detrimental effects on health. So the single most important exercise for anyone unfit and on a diet is moderate walking – about 20 minutes per day. But this does not imply that you should walk in the morning (before work) or in the evening (after work). On the contrary, you should *incorporate* exercise into your working day (and in this we certainly include mothers at home who work much harder in their occupation than any other of which we are aware!).

Park the car, or alight from the bus, with a further 10 minute walk to your place of work and you have automatically completed your walking regime. Or walk to lunch 10 minutes from the office. A round trip will automatically complete the walking component of the exercise programme for the day.

But walking is not the only part of the exercise regime that can be easily incorporated into your working day, irrespective of how busy your schedule. The important point is to use the myriad free moments in your day – every day – to maximum effect.

You may not consider that you have any free time during the working day, but you do! For a moment, just consider how much time you spend sitting at your desk, or even waiting for a meal to cook in the kitchen! All this time, which would otherwise be completely wasted, can be effectively utilised within your daily exercise regime, because this is a *practical* programme designed to fit around *your* lifestyle – not the other way around. And because the exercise programme fits your lifestyle (as with the diet) it is easy to perform on a regular basis and is therefore bound to be successful.

This exercise programme will combine isotonic and isometric exercises, the principles of which are explained in detail in *The New High Protein Diet* but the basis is simply as follows.

Isotonic exercises are the usual form of exercise which you immediately associate with the term exercise. This involves movement of the muscles, as in walking or aerobics.

Isometric exercises do not involve any movement or any special equipment whatsoever, so they are ideally suited to an exercise programme that can be performed almost anywhere. How can you possibly exercise without moving? Quite simply, because you contract your muscles against an immovable object, such as a table or doorway. Let us provide a simple example. Sit on a dining chair at a normal table, extend your arms in front of

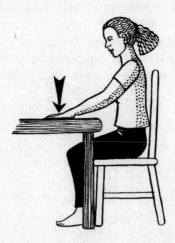

you and place your hands palm downwards on the table.

Take a deep breath and, sitting perfectly still, press your hands down on the table surface and keep pressing constantly for 6–8 seconds, then relax. This is a strengthening exercise for the upper back muscles and you will have felt the muscle tension in your upper back during the exercise. Performing this simple exercise 4–5 days per week will result in considerable strengthening of the upper back muscles. And, as you can appreciate, this can be easily performed at home or at a desk in the office.

Now that you can appreciate how simply and easily an effective exercise programme can be incorporated into your daily life, we can describe exercises which can be easily adapted to virtually every busy lifestyle and be incorporated into the working day in such a manner that they effectively take up no dedicated time whatsoever.

We will assume that you are exercising the muscles of your lower limbs by walking 20 minutes per day, the isotonic component of the programme. The following exercises are designed primarily for the upper body i.e. waist upwards.

Neck exercises

Always commence your exercise programme with neck exercises. These are almost always forgotten during a typical exercise regime but they are most important to prevent subsequent arthritis affecting the vertebrae of the upper back. *Isometric* exercises to strengthen the muscles of the neck were described in *The New High Protein Diet*. The following are *isotonic* exercises which improve the mobility of the neck and help to prevent neck pain and weakness of the muscles of the arms from constriction of the nerves (cervical spondylosis) which is common in later life.

Warning: Do not perform neck exercises if you have any medical history of neck injury or problems, or if you have any evidence of reduced circulation to the brain. Always consult your personal physician before commencing any form of exercise regime.

There are four basic movements required to exercise the full range of movement of the neck.

Forward flexion and extension

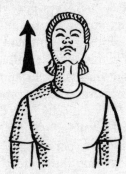

Bend your head forward until your chin touches your chest then lift your head backwards as far as you can. *Do not force the movement*. You may find that your neck movements are quite stiff, especially if you have not performed neck exercises for many years (or perhaps never!). The flexion of neck movements will gradually increase over a period of a few weeks with regular exercise.

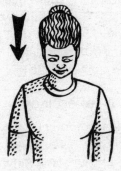

Repeat the movement 5 times.

Lateral flexion and extension

Whilst looking straight ahead, bend your neck to the left side and try to place your left ear on your left shoulder. *Do not force the movement*.

Then lift your head to the upright position and try to

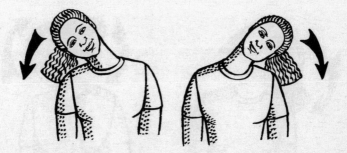

place your right ear on your right shoulder. Repeat the movement 5 times.

Lateral rotation

With your head in the upright position, turn your head to the right as far as you are able to *comfortably achieve*, then turn your head in the opposite direction to the left. Repeat the movement 5 times.

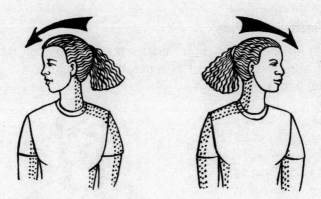

Circular rotation

Tilt your head backwards until the back of your head touches your upper back then rotate your head around to the left until your chin touches your chest. Continue the movement to the right until you have completed a complete rotation of the neck and the

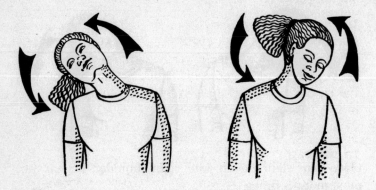

back of your head is again resting on the back of your neck. Repeat the movement 5 times.

Perform the opposite rotation by tilting your head backwards until the back of your head touches your upper back, then rotate your head to the right until you complete a rotation. Once again, repeat the exercise 5 times.

Chest exercise

Mild exercise of the chest muscles is very important for cosmetic reasons as well as general improvement in condition. For a man, a firm chest is very desirable. For a woman, firming the chest muscles improves and tones the bustline without unsightly muscle contours.

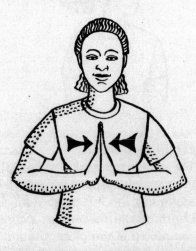

Exercises for the chest muscles can be performed almost anywhere. We will describe two of the most common situations: a) In the office/at home b) In the car

In the office/at home
Clasp both hands together in front of your chest with elbows bent. Take a deep breath in and hold, then press both palms together as firmly as you can; hold the contraction for 6–8 seconds whilst holding your breath, and relax.

In the car
This exercise can only be performed whilst sitting in the car when the car is stationary for a few minutes.

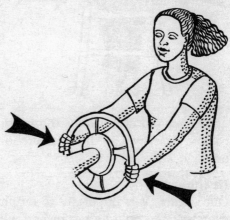

Sit upright in the driving seat, extend your arms to the front, place both hands on the outer edges of the steering wheel and grasp the wheel tightly. Take a deep breath in and hold, then press both hands together as firmly as you can, hold the contraction for 6-8 seconds and relax.

Upper back exercise

The upper back muscles balance the chest muscles; if you exercise one group of muscles more than the other, a muscle imbalance occurs so it is important to always exercise both at the same session. There are two exercises for the upper back muscles that are very important.

Once again, we will describe two of the commonest situations: in the office and in the car.

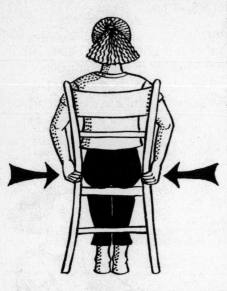

In the office/at home

Sit upright in a straight-backed chair, place both hands behind your back and grasp the outer edges of the chair firmly. Take a deep breath in and hold then press both hands together as firmly as you can. Hold the contraction for 6–8 seconds and relax.

The second exercise for the muscles of the upper back is described in the introduction to this chapter on page 293.

In the car

Once again, it is important to emphasise that these exercises can only be performed whilst sitting in the car when the car is stationary for a few minutes. *Never* perform these exercises while you are actually driving.

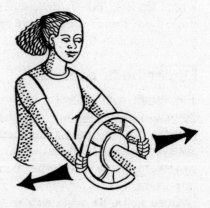

Sit upright in the driving seat, extend your arms to the front and place both hands on the outer edges of the steering wheel and grasp the wheel tightly.

Take a deep breath in and hold, then try to pull your hands *away* from one another in an outwards direction, hold the contraction for 6–8 seconds and relax.

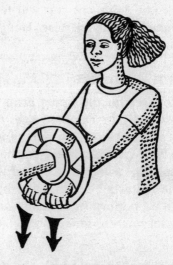

The second movement exercises the broad upper back muscles. Sitting upright in the driving seat, extend your arms to the front, place both hands on the lower margin of the steering wheel and grasp the wheel tightly. Take a deep breath in and hold then try to push your hands *downwards* towards the floor, hold the contraction for 6-8 seconds and relax.

Shoulder exercise

This exercise can be easily performed in the office, at home or in a stationary car.

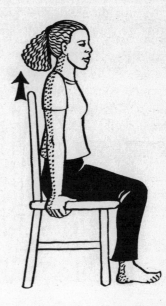

Sit upright on a straight-back chair (or seat in the car). Place both arms by your sides and grasp each side of the seat of the chair tightly. Take a deep breath in and hold, then keeping your arms straight by your sides attempt to shrug your shoulders. Your shoulders

299

will not move but you will feel the muscle tension created by the exercise. Hold the tension for 8–10 seconds and *relax*.

Arm exercises

Exercises for the upper arms have been described previously in *The New High Protein Diet*, however these exercises form part of a comprehensive upper body 'workout' and can be adapted to virtually every situation, whether in the office, at home or in the car. The following demonstrate how this form of exercise can be performed virtually anywhere. We begin by increasing the tone of the *flexor* muscles (biceps).

In the office/at home

These exercises utilise a desk or table. Use a *heavy* table (or desk) as you may find that you lift the table as your strength increases – and it will definitely increase with this simple exercise programme.

Sit upright about 20–25 cm from the desk. Place your arms by your sides then bend the elbows at a right

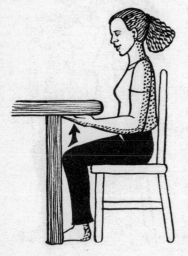

angle. Place your hands under the desk, palms facing upwards against the under surface of the desk.

Take a deep breath in and hold, press *upwards* with both hands as if attempting to lift the desk. Hold the tension for 8–10 seconds and relax.

In the car

Sit upright about 20–25 cm from the steering wheel. Place your arms by your sides then bend the elbows

300

at a right angle. Grasp the lower rim of the steering wheel tightly, palms facing upwards. Take a deep breath in and hold, press *upwards* with both hands as if attempting to lift the steering wheel. Hold the tension for 8-10 seconds and relax.

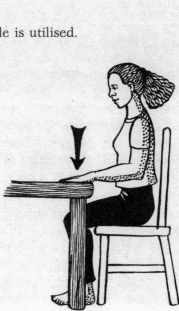

Obviously, having exercised the *flexor* (or biceps) muscles of the arm (which bend the arm), we have to exercise the *extensor* (or triceps) muscles (which straighten the arm) to maintain a muscular balance.

In the office/at home
Once again a desk or table is utilised.

Sit upright about 20–25 cm from the desk. Place your arms by your sides then bend the elbows at a right angle. Place both hands on the desk top, palms facing downwards. Take a deep breath in and hold, press *down* with both hands as if attempting to press the desk to the floor. Hold the tension for 8–10 seconds and relax.

In the car

Sit upright about 20–25 cm from the steering wheel. Place your arms by your sides then bend the elbows at a right angle. Grasp the lower rim of the steering wheel tightly, palms facing down. Take a deep breath in and hold, press *down* with both hands as if attempting to press the steering wheel to the floor. Hold the tension for 8–10 seconds and relax.

Abdominal exercise

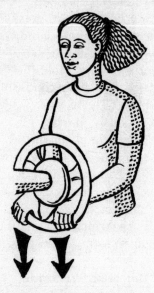

Increasing the tone of the muscles of the abdomen (tummy) is remarkably easily performed in virtually every situation. It is important to emphasise that when you have not performed strenuous exercise on a semi-regular basis for a long time, you should *never* over-exercise or over-exert yourself initially. This is the mistake which most people make when commencing a weight loss programme and it is very dangerous. It is particularly common in relation to the abdominal muscles where you are encouraged to believe that strenuous abdominal exercise will lead to a 'six-pack' for a man or a slim waist for a woman. Nothing could be further from the truth! If you have not exercised the abdominal muscles for years (or possibly never) they are very underdeveloped and wasted and you will only succeed in causing pain and muscle damage by overexertion. The following exercise is the safest for those who have not previously performed abdominal exercises, can be performed

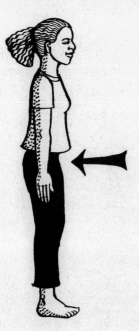

literally anywhere, and has no potential side-effects.

Standing upright, breathe out almost completely. 'Pull in' your abdominal muscles and hold the contraction for 6–8 seconds then relax. Repeat the exercise 4–5 times per day, but leaving at least 30 minutes between each contraction.

Index

amino acids 5, 16
arthritis, premature 9
asparagus
  Asparagus with Wild Rocket and
    Mint Sauce 260
  Chargrilled Basil Pesto Salmon with
    Asparagus 225–6
  Steak with Asparagus Purée 171–2
Atkins Diet 47–8
aubergine, Gammon and Aubergine
  with Herbs 210–11
avocado
  Avocado on Toast 104
  Avocado with Bocconcini Cheese 146
  Chicken and Wild Rocket Salad
    265–6
  Chicken with Mayonnaise and
    Avocado open sandwich 155
  Smoked Trout with Avocado 163–4
  for breakfast 78–9
  health benefits 69

bacon
  Lettuce and Tomato open sandwich
    157–8
  Mushrooms with Bacon 102–3
  for breakfast 91–3
Balsamic Vinaigrette 274
basil
  Basil Bocconcini with Spinach
    254–5
  Basil Pesto Sauce 275
  Chargrilled Basil Pesto Salmon with
    Asparagus 225–6
  Cherry Tomatoes with Basil and
    Coriander 262
  Egg Mayonnaise with Fresh Basil
    and Chives 144–5
  Grilled Ham with Mozzarella, Basil
    and Cherry Tomatoes 215–16
  Meatballs with Tomato and Basil
    Sauce 199–200
  Salmon with Bocconcini and Basil
    211
  Steak with Cherry Tomatoes, Basil
    and Coriander 220
  Tuna Mayonnaise with Basil and
    Coriander 146–7
  Whiting with Scrambled Eggs and
    Basil 100–1
beef
  Balti Beef 215
  Beef Bolognaise with Mushrooms
    187–9
  Beef Jalfrezi Curry with Peppers
    190–1

Chilli Con Carne 186–7
  Meatballs with Tomato and Basil
    Sauce 199–200
  Roast Beef and Pickle 147
  Salsa Steak open sandwich 158–9
  Sesame Beef with Ginger and
    Lemongrass 206–7
  Steak with Asparagus Purée 171–2
  Steak with Cherry Tomatoes, Basil
    and Coriander 220
  Steak with Spinach and Caramelised
    Onions 189–90
  Swedish Meatballs with Herbs
    216–17
  Sweet and Sour Beef with
    Mangetout 208–10
  Thai Koftas with Mango Raita 203–4
baking (in a casserole) 61
  for breakfast 81
  frying 60–1
  grilling 61
  microwaving 62
  roasting 61–2
  stir-frying 60–1
  stock items 42
  what to buy 59
bistro meals
  breakfast 104–5
  dinner 238–40
  lunch 173–5
body fat
  effects of carbohydrates on 8–9
  regulation by insulin 8–9
Bok Choi with Cinnamon 259
bread, nutritional value 11
breakfast 73–110
  and fat burning 20–1
  bistro 104–5
  Burger King 107
  continental 77–84
  cooked 84–104
  effects of carbohydrates 74–5
  importance of 20–1, 73–4
  McDonald's 107
  take-away food 105–10
  use of the microwave oven 76–7
  without carbohydrates 75–6
broccoli
  Broccoli with Garlic and Spring
    Onions 261
  Chicken Korma with Mangetout and
    Broccoli 195–7
  Lamb Tikka Masala with Broccoli
    197–8
Brussels Sprouts with Orange and
Lemon Butter Sauce 260–1

Burger King 115
  adapting to low-carb 135-7
  breakfasts 107
  items to be excluded 140

calcium 5, 14-15
carbohydrate addiction 37
carbohydrate content, on food labels. 23-4
carbohydrates
  and obesity 9
  effects on insulin levels 8-9
  eliminating from diet 7-13
  'good' and 'bad' 10-12
  guidelines for restricting 36-7
  refined 9-10
  substituting alternatives 22-3
cheese
  Avocado with Bocconcini Cheese 146
  Basil Bocconcini with Spinach 254-5
  Basil Pesto Sauce 275
  Gammon and Aubergine with Herbs 210-11
  Greek Salad 148-9
  Grilled Ham with Mozzarella, Basil and Cherry Tomatoes 215-16
  Haddock with Grilled Leerdammer 99-100
  Mozzarella and Tomato Omelette 220-1
  Pepper and Herb Frittata 257-8
  Peppered Smoked Ham with Spinach and Ricotta 219
  Port Salut, Courgettes and Chives Salad 151-2
  Roast Ham with Leerdammer Cheese and Mustard 145
  Salmon with Bocconcini and Basil 211
  Spinach and Emmental Crêpes 169-70
  Three Cheese Salad 264
  Toasted Cheese 93-5
  for breakfast 77-8, 93-5
  stock items 42
  varieties 94-5
Cherry Tomatoes with Basil and Coriander 262
chicken
  Balti Chicken 214-15
  Chicken and Wild Rocket Salad 265-6
  Chicken Breast with Chilli Sauce 143-4
  Chicken Korma with Mangetout and Broccoli 195-7
  Chicken Satay with Lime 192-3
  Chicken with Curry and Herb Sauce 149-50

Chicken with Mayonnaise and Avocado open sandwich 155
Hot-and-Spicy Chicken Drumsticks with Baby Spinach Leaves 160-1
Spicy Chicken Drumsticks 184
Thai Chicken with Lemongrass and Ginger 193-5
baking 64
for breakfast 81-2
frying 63, 64
microwaving 64
roasting 64
stir-frying 63
what to buy 62
children, development of diabetes 12-13
chillies *see also* peppers (capsicums)
  Chilli Con Carne 186-7
  Chilli Prawns 224-5
  Chilli Vegetables 254
  health benefits 111
Chinese restaurants 244-5
Chinese take-away food 115, 139
chromium 2
continental sausages, for breakfast 79-80
cooking equipment 25, 26-30
  microwave 25, 26-30
crêpe-maker 25
crêpes
  Hoisin Duck 168
  Prawn Mayonnaise 169
  Savoury 166-70
  Spinach and Emmental 169-70
cucumber
  Cucumber Raita 276
  Gazpacho Salad 267-8
  Radicchio and Cucumber Salad 267

delicatessen
  lunches 127-9
  Marks and Spencer 119-25
  supermarket 119-25
  take-away sandwiches 109-10
diabetes 9
  and chromium 2
  and diet 12-13, 51-2
  Type 1 51
  Type 2 51-2
diet (New High Protein)
  balance and nutrition 13-17
  basic principles for health and success 7-31
  dieter's commitment to 30-1
  Frequently Asked Questions 47-52
  financial cost of 17-19
  general guidelines 35-40
  health aspects 47-52
  planning ahead 21
  stock of essential foods 38-44

summary of principles 30
dinner 177–248
  bistro 238–40
  Chinese restaurants 244–5
  French cuisine 242–4
  Indian restaurants 245–7
  Italian restaurants 240–1
  quick–and–easy dinner at home
    181–218
  ready–prepared meals at home
    226–37
  really fast suppers 218–26
  restaurant meals 237–48
  Thai restaurants 247–8
dressings
  Balsamic Vinaigrette 274
  French vinaigrette 273
  ingredients for 41–2
  Lemon Vinaigrette 274

eggs
  Basil Bocconcini with Spinach 254–5
  Boiled Eggs 85
  Egg Mayonnaise with Fresh Basil
    and Chives 144–5
  Eggs Benedict 217–18
  Fried Eggs 90–1
  Ham, Eggs and Chives open
    sandwich 155–6
  Mozzarella and Tomato Omelette
    220–1
  Omelette 87–9
  Pepper and Herb Frittata 257–8
  Poached Eggs 89–90
  Prawn Omelette 201–2
  Scrambled Eggs 85–7
  Smoked Haddock with Poached Eggs
    101–2
  Spicy Scrambled Eggs 207–8
  Whiting with Scrambled Eggs and
    Basil 100–1
  for breakfast 82, 85–91
  quick cooking methods 67
  stock items 42
  what to buy 67
essential nutrients 15–17
exercise
  and osteoarthritis 290
  choosing the correct type 289–93
  heart attack risk 290–1
  isometric 292
  isotonic 292
  jogging 290
  pain during 290–1
  to fit your lifestyle 291–2 *see also*
    exercise plan
  weight training 290
exercise plan 289–303
  abdominal exercise 302–3
  arm exercises 300–2

chest exercise 296–7
neck exercises 293–6
shoulder exercise 299–300
upper back exercises 292–3, 297–9
walking 291

fast food, relative cost of 18–19
fat burning, and diet 20–1, 22
fats, in the diet 8, 50–1
fatty acids, essential 16–17
fish *see also* shellfish
  Chargrilled Basil Pesto Salmon with
    Asparagus 225–6
  Chargrilled Madras Sardines with
    Crème Fraîche 172
  Cod with Orange Sauce 170–1
  Haddock with Grilled Leerdammer
    99–100
  Haddock with Herbs 162–3
  Kippers 96–7
  Mint Cod with Spinach 185–6
  Peppered Smoked Mackerel with
    Spinach in Butter Sauce 223
  Plaice with Olives 213–14
  Salmon with Bocconcini and Basil
    211
  Salmon with Crème Fraîche 147–8
  Salmon with Lime Butter Sauce and
    Watercress 182–3
  Salmon with Wild Rocket and Mint
    Sauce 221–2
  Sardines with Herbs 100
  Smoked Haddock with Poached Eggs
    101–2
  Smoked Trout with Avocado 163–4
  Trout with Coriander and Lemon
    Butter Sauce 97–8
  Tuna Mayonnaise open sandwich
    156–7
  Tuna Mayonnaise with Basil and
    Coriander 146–7
  Tuna with Spinach and Basil 165–6
  Whiting with Herbs 98–9
  Whiting with Scrambled Eggs and
    Basil 100–1
  baking 66
  for breakfast 95–102
  for breakfast (pre–cooked) 82–3
  frozen 43, 65–6
  frying 66
  grilling 66–7
  health benefits 5, 43
  microwaving 67
  pre–cooked and packaged 65, 82–3
  raw 66
  shellfish 43
  steaming 66
  stock items 42–3
  tinned 43, 65
  what to buy 65

folic acid 111
food labels 23–4, 120
food shopping online 39
foods
  essential items 38–44
  excluded during the weight-loss
    phase 38
  quick preparation methods 55–67
  restricted 35–6, 38
  unrestricted 35, 37–8
French cuisine 242–4
French vinaigrette 273
Frequently-Asked Questions 47–52
fruit 43
  carbohydrate content of different
    types 83–4
  for breakfast 83–4

gammon
  Gammon and Aubergine with Herbs
    210–11
  Gammon Steaks with Balsamic
    Vinegar 163
  Gammon Steaks with Honey 200–1
  for breakfast 91–3
Gazpacho Salad 267–8
Greek Salad 148–9

ham
  Eggs Benedict 217–18
  Grilled Ham with Mozzarella, Basil
    and Cherry Tomatoes 215–16
  Ham, Eggs and Chives open
    sandwich 155–6
  Peppered Smoked Ham with
    Spinach and Ricotta 219
  Roast Ham with Leerdammer
    Cheese and Mustard 145
  for breakfast 79
heart
  dangers of strenuous exercise 290–1
  effects of low-carbohydrate diet 52
heart disease 9
  and diet 52
herbs
  essential items 41
  fresh 56
high blood pressure 9
Hoisin Vegetables 255–6
hormones, functions in the body 7–9
hunger
  as cause of failed diets 143
  avoiding 19–21, 22
  while dieting 13

Indian food, choosing ready-prepared
  meals 235–7
Indian restaurants 245–7
Indian take-away food 115, 139
insulin
  levels on low-calorie diets 14
  regulation of body fat 8–9
insulin production, and exercise 289
insulin resistance 12
  and Type 2 diabetes 51–2
isometric exercise 292
isotonic exercise 292
Italian restaurants 240–1

jogging 290

Kentucky Fried Chicken 115
  adapting to low-carb 137
  items to be excluded 141
kidneys, effects of high-protein diet
  49–50
kitchen equipment 25, 26–30
  microwave ovens 25, 26–30

lamb
  Lamb Tikka Masala with Broccoli
    197–8
  Swedish Meatballs with Herbs
    216–17
  Tandoori Lamb with Cucumber
    Raita 165
  baking (in a casserole) 61
  frying 60–1
  grilling 61
  microwaving 62
  ready cooked 60
  roasting 61–2
  stir-frying 60–1
  stock items 42
  what to buy 59
leeks, Baby Leeks in Lemon Butter
  Sauce 262–3
Lemon Vinaigrette 274
low-calorie diets 7
  and high insulin levels 14
  and hunger 13, 19–20
  and osteoporosis 50
  nutritional deficiencies 13–15
  problems caused by 8
low-calorie foods, avoiding 226–7
low-carbohydrate diet 7, 8 *see also*
  New High Protein Diet
  effects on the heart 52
low-fat diets 8
  and osteoporosis 50
low-fat foods, avoiding 226–7
lunch 111–75
  adapting take-away food 115–17
  at home 160–72
  bistro 173–5
  packed 141–60
  take-away (cold) 117–32
  take-away (hot) 132–41
lycopene 177

Mango Raita 275
Marks and Spencer
  delicatessen foods 119–25
  take-away section 117–19
mayonnaise
  Chicken with Mayonnaise and
    Avocado open sandwich 155
  Egg Mayonnaise with Fresh Basil
    and Chives 144–5
  Prawn Mayonnaise Crêpes 169
  Prawn Mayonnaise open sandwich
    156
  Spicy Mayonnaise 164–5
  Tuna Mayonnaise open sandwich
    156–7
  Tuna Mayonnaise with Basil and
    Coriander 146–7
McDonald's 38, 115
  adapting to low-carb 133–5
  breakfasts 107
  items to be excluded 140
meal plan, examples for one month
    279–85
meats see also bacon; beef; ham;
    lamb; pork
  Salami Salad open sandwich 159
  breakfast (cold meats) 79–81
  cooking methods 60–2
  ready cooked 60
  stock items 42
  what to buy 59
microwave cooking 23, 25, 26–30
  cost of 28
microwave cookware 25, 28–9
microwave oven
  for cooked breakfasts 84–5 see also
    individual recipes
  how it works 26–7
  power rating 29–30
  what it can do 27–8
  what it can't do 28
milk, calcium levels 14–15
minerals 16, 17
mushrooms
  Beef Bolognaise with Mushrooms
    187–9
  Mushrooms with Bacon 102–3
  Tomatoes with Mushrooms 103
  for breakfast 102–3

New High Protein Diet
  balance and nutrition 13–17
  basic principles for health and
    success 7–31
  dieter's commitment to 30–1
  Frequently-Asked Questions 47–52
  financial cost of 17–19
  general guidelines 35–40
  health aspects 47–52
  nutrient provision 49

  planning ahead 21
  stock of essential foods 38–44
  summary of principles 30
nutrients, essential 15–17
nutrition, elements of a healthy diet
    13–17
nutritional label, importance of
    reading 24–4, 120
nuts, stock items 43

obesity, and carbohydrate
    consumption 9
oils, for cooking and dressings 41
olive oil, health benefits 269
olives
  Plaice with Olives 213–14
  health benefits 213
omega-3 fatty acids 5, 16
omega-6 fatty acids 16–17
open sandwiches 153–9
  container for 153
osteoporosis
  and diet 14–15
  and the New High Protein Diet 50
  causes of 50

packed lunch 141–60
pasta dishes, to be excluded 232–4
pepper, black 2
peppercorns, whole 43
peppers (capsicums) see also chillies
  Beef Jalfrezi Curry with Peppers
    190–1
  Gazpacho Salad 267–8
  Hoisin Vegetables 255–6
  Peperonata 256
  Pepper and Herb Frittata 257–8
  Rocket and Tofu Salad 266
  Thai Chicken with Lemongrass and
    Ginger 193–5
  Turkey Bolognaise with Peppers
    204–6
  health benefits 111
pizza, relative cost of 18–19
pork
  Balti Pork 215
  Pork Chops with Brussels Sprouts
    and Citrus Butter Sauce 222–3
  Swedish Meatballs with Herbs
    216–17
  baking (in a casserole) 61
  frying 60–1
  grilling 61
  microwaving 62
  ready cooked 60
  roasting 61–2
  stir-frying 60–1
  stock items 42
  what to buy 59
potassium 69

poultry
  Duck with Plum Sauce 185
  Hoisin Duck Crêpes 168
  Peking Duck 212
  cooking methods 63–4
  for breakfast 81–2
  stock items 42
  what to buy 62
prawns *see* shellfish
protein
  effects of high levels in the diet
    48–9, 49–50
  in the body 16
  in the diet 8

Radicchio and Cucumber Salad 267
Radish and Mint Salad 265
restaurant meals 237–48
rice dishes, to be excluded 232–4
Rocket and Tofu Salad 266

salad boxes to take away 127, 129
salad lunchbox meals 142–52
salads 263–8 *see also* dressings
  Chicken and Wild Rocket Salad
    265–6
  Crab Salad open sandwich 158
  Crispy Herb Salad 263
  Gazpacho Salad 267–8
  Greek Salad 148–9
  Port Salut, Courgettes and Chives
    Salad 151–2
  Radicchio and Cucumber Salad 267
  Radish and Mint Salad 265
  Rocket and Tofu Salad 266
  Salami Salad open sandwich 159
  Three Cheese Salad 264
  Tikka Masala Salad 263–4
  essential items 40–1
  ready-prepared 40–1, 58
salami *see also* hams; meats
  Salami Salad open sandwich 159
  for breakfast 80–1
salmon
  Chargrilled Basil Pesto Salmon with
    Asparagus 225–6
  Salmon with Bocconcini and Basil
    211
  Salmon with Crème Fraîche 147–8
  Salmon with Lime Butter Sauce and
    Watercress 182–3
  Salmon with Wild Rocket and Mint
    Sauce 221–2
  health benefits 211
  microwave cooking 23
  relative cost of 18–19
sandwiches
  open sandwich recipes 153–9
  take-away 107–10, 125–7, 129–30
sauces 41–2, 274–6

Basil Pesto Sauce 275
Cucumber Raita 276
Mango Raita 275
Tomato Sauce 274–5
Wild Rocket and Mint Sauce 276
Savoury Crêpes 166–70
seafood *see* fish; shellfish
seeds, stock items 43
selenium 177
shellfish 43 *see also* fish
  Chilli Prawns 224–5
  Crab Salad open sandwich 158
  Prawn Mayonnaise Crêpes 169
  Prawn Mayonnaise open sandwich
    156
  Prawn Omelette 201–2
  Spicy Prawns with Rocket 164–5
  Tiger Prawns with Chilli and
    Coriander Vinaigrette 150–1
  Tiger Prawns with Lemon and
    Coriander Vinaigrette 151
  frozen 65–6
  microwaving 67
  pre-cooked and packaged 65
  raw 66
  steaming 66
  stir-frying 66
  what to buy 65
shish kebabs 132
shopping, planning ahead 21
spices, stock items 43
spinach
  Basil Bocconcini with Spinach
    254–5
  Mint Cod with Rocket and Spinach
    185–6
  Peppered Smoked Ham with
    Spinach and Ricotta 219
  Peppered Smoked Mackerel with
    Spinach in Butter Sauce 223
  Spinach and Emmental Crêpes
    169–70
  Spinach with Butter Sauce 259
  Steak with Spinach and Caramelised
    Onions 189–90
  health benefits 219
steaming vegetables 25
stir-frying 25
  Stir-Fried Vegetables with Black
    Bean Sauce 258
  beef 60–1
  chicken 63
  lamb 60–1
  pork 60–1
  shellfish 66
  turkey 63
  vegetables 56–7, 58
stock cubes 42
stocks (flavourings) 42
Subway sandwich outlets 129–30

supermarkets
  choosing ready-prepared foods
    226-37
  delicatessen foods 119-25
  foods to be avoided 130-2
  take-away section 117-19

take-away foods
  breakfasts 105-10
  foods to be avoided (cold) 130-2
  foods to be avoided (hot) 138-41
  lunch, cold 117-32
  lunch, hot 132-41
  salad boxes 127, 129
  sandwiches 107-10, 125-7, 129-30
Teriyaki Tofu 256-7
Thai restaurants 247-8
Tiger Prawns with Chilli and
  Coriander Vinaigrette 150-1
Tiger Prawns with Lemon and
  Coriander Vinaigrette 151
Tikka Masala Salad 263-4
tofu
  Rocket and Tofu Salad 266
  Teriyaki Tofu 256-7
tomatoes
  Bacon, Lettuce and Tomato open
    sandwich 157-8
  Cherry Tomatoes with Basil and
    Coriander 262
  Grilled Ham with Mozzarella, Basil
    and Cherry Tomatoes 215-16
  Mozzarella and Tomato Omelette
    220-1
  Steak with Cherry Tomatoes, Basil
    and Coriander 220
  Tomato Sauce 274-5
  Tomatoes with Mushrooms 103
  Turkey in Cherry Tomato and Chilli
    Sauce 202-3
  for breakfast 78
  health benefits 177
turkey
  Bombay Turkey Breast with
    Watercress and Rocket Salad 223-4
  Swedish Meatballs with Herbs
    216-17
  Tikka Masala Salad 263-4
  Turkey Bolognaise with Peppers
    204-6
  Turkey in Cherry Tomato and Chilli
    Sauce 202-3
  Turkey Teriyaki 198-9
  baking 64
  for breakfast 81-2
  frying 63, 64
  microwaving 64
  roasting 64

stir-frying 63
what to buy 62
vegetarian dishes 254-63 see also
  salads and individual vegetables
  Asparagus with Wild Rocket and
    Mint Sauce 260
  Baby Leeks in Lemon Butter Sauce
    262-3
  Basil Bocconcini with Spinach 254-5
  Bok Choi with Cinnamon 259
  Broccoli with Garlic and Spring
    Onions 261
  Brussels Sprouts with Orange and
    Lemon Butter Sauce 260-1
  Cherry Tomatoes with Basil and
    Coriander 262
  Chilli Vegetables 254
  Hoisin Vegetables 255-6
  Peperonata 256
  Pepper and Herb Frittata 257-8
  Spinach with Butter Sauce 259
  Stir-Fried Vegetables with Black
    Bean Sauce 258
  Teriyaki Tofu 256-7
  Watercress with Ginger 261-2
vegetables
  boiling 59
  cooking methods 56-9
  essential items 40-1
  frozen 55-6, 57-8
  microwaving 59
  quickly prepared side dishes 253
  ready-prepared 40-1, 56-7, 232
  steaming 58-9
  stir-frying 56-7, 58
  tinned 55, 57
  what to buy 55-6
vitamin A 111, 177
vitamin B$_1$ 102, 111
vitamin B$_2$ 69, 102
vitamin B$_6$ 69
vitamin B$_{12}$, in the diet 15
vitamin C 111, 177
vitamin D 5, 14-15
vitamin E 69
vitamins 16, 17

Watercress with Ginger 261-2
weight maintenance 12
weight reduction, on a healthy diet
  15-16
weight training 290
Wild Rocket and Mint Sauce 276
willpower 13

yoghurt
  Cucumber Raita 276
  Mango Raita 275

ALSO AVAILABLE FROM VERMILION
BY DR CHARLES CLARK

The New High Protein Diet	0091884268	£7.99
The New High Protein Diet Cookbook	0091889707	£7.99
The Ultimate Diet Counter	0091889715	£3.99

FREE POSTAGE AND PACKING
Overseas customers allow £2.00 per paperback

ORDER:

By phone: 01624 677237

By post: Random House Books
c/o Bookpost
PO Box 29
Douglas
Isle of Man IM991BQ

By fax: 01624 670923

By email: bookshop@enterprise.net

Cheques (payable to Bookpost) and credit cards accepted

Prices and availability subject to change without notice.
Allow 28 days for delivery.

When placing your order, please mention if you do not
wish to receive any additional information.

www.randomhouse.co.uk